D1417754

EPIDEMICS AND SOCIETY™

CHOLERA

DIANE BAILEY

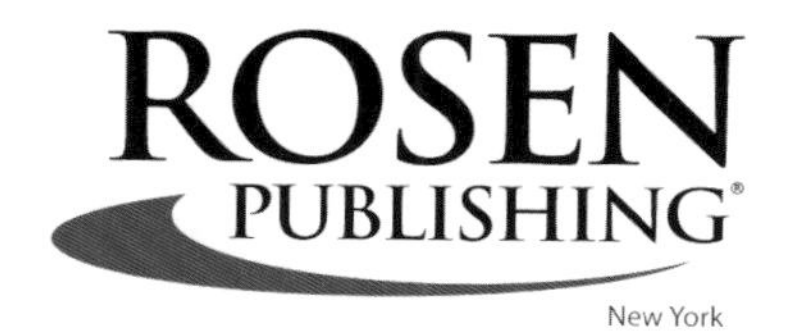

Published in 2011 by The Rosen Publishing Group, Inc.
29 East 21st Street, New York, NY 10010

First Edition

Library of Congress Cataloging-in-Publication Data

Bailey, Diane, 1966 –
Cholera / Diane Bailey. — 1st ed.
p. cm. — (Epidemics and society)
Includes bibliographical references and index.
ISBN 978-1-4358-9437-2 (library binding)
1. Cholera—Popular works. I. Title.
RC126.B28 2011
614.5'14—dc22

2009046610

Manufactured in the United States of America

CPSIA Compliance Information: Batch #S10YA: For further information, contact Rosen Publishing, New York, New York, at 1-800-237-9932.

On the cover: *Vibrio cholerae*, the bacteria that cause cholera.

CONTENTS

INTRODUCTION

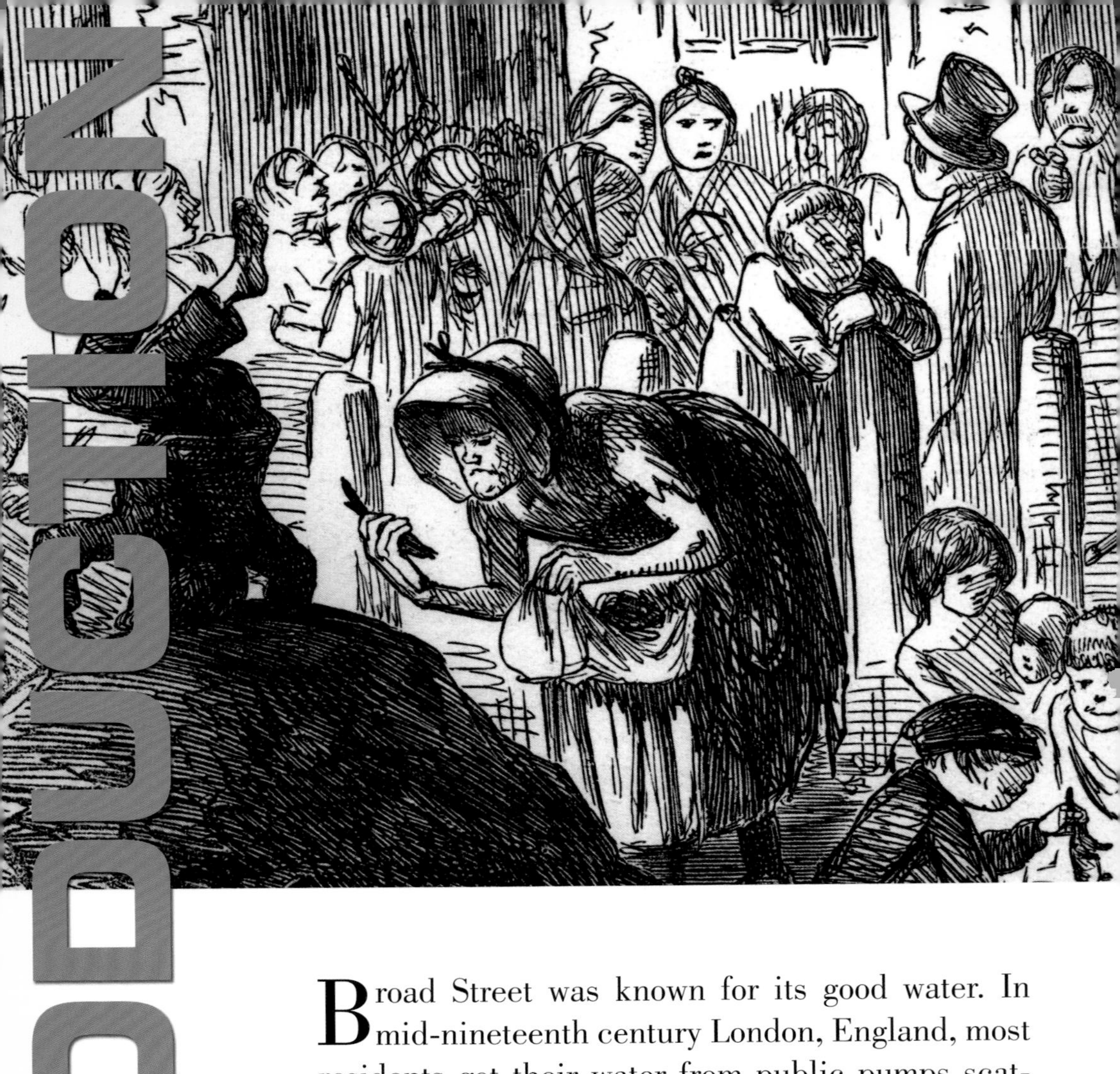

Broad Street was known for its good water. In mid-nineteenth century London, England, most residents got their water from public pumps scattered throughout the city. At most of the pumps, the water wasn't always very good. But Broad Street was different. People went out of their way to go there. Water from the Broad Street pump looked clean and tasted good.

But in September 1854, that same water also killed. It hid bacteria that caused cholera.

The cholera outbreak in the fall of 1854 was fast and furious. People suffered from cramps, vomiting, and diarrhea. Death came to hundreds. The

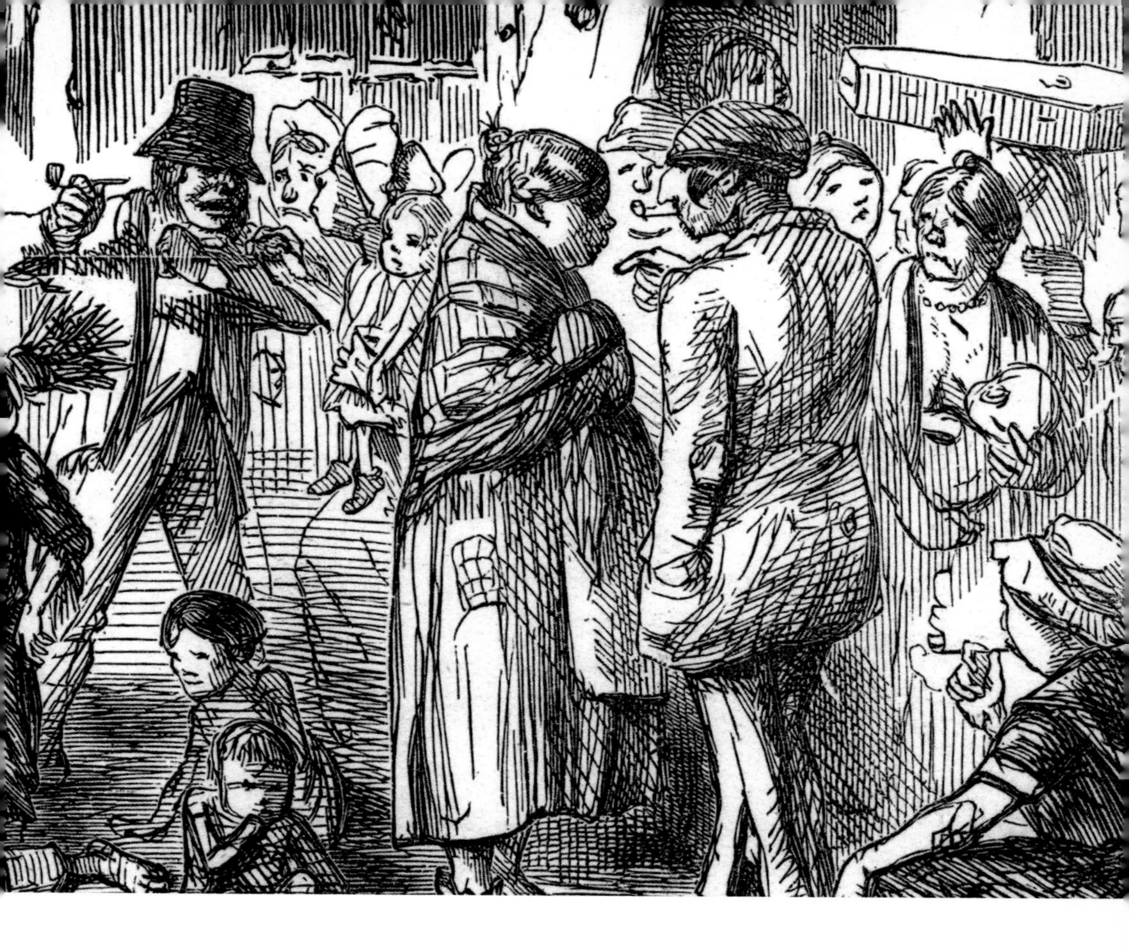

In crowded cities, piles of garbage in the streets helped spread cholera. In the background, a casket being carried away is a reminder of the thousands of deaths the disease caused.

disease spread from house to house around the Golden Square area of London.

A doctor named John Snow was positive there was some link between these people—something that the rest of London didn't share. That something, he was sure, was water. To prove his theory, Snow began recording all the cholera cases he ran across. Then he made a map of this area in London and marked where each case occurred.

When he finished, he saw that most of the victims that died lived within blocks of the Broad Street pump. Snow set out to interview the families of the victims. One by one, they told him the same thing: they got their water from the Broad Street pump.

Snow was convinced that the outbreak was tied to the pump. His next step was to try to stop it. He told the health board what he had found and asked it to remove the handle from the pump. Members of the board thought Snow's theory was ridiculous. However, they had no better solution. They agreed to remove the handle.

By that time, a week had passed. The outbreak was probably over anyway. Underground, without any air or light, the cholera bacteria had probably died. Still, the question remained of what had caused the outbreak in the first place. Further investigation led to the Lewis family. They lived right next to the pump. A baby in the family had come down with cholera. The mother had thrown the baby's diarrhea into a nearby cesspool (a place for wastewater and sewage). Unfortunately, the cesspool leaked. Cholera bacteria in the baby's waste contaminated the clean water source next to it—the Broad Street pump.

By the end of that week in September, more than six hundred people had died. But there was another case yet to come. The outbreak had started with the Lewis baby, and now it came back to that family. The baby's father got sick. His wife probably threw his waste into the same leaky cesspool. But now there was no handle on the Broad Street pump and, therefore, no way for cholera bacteria to reach more people. John Snow's simple solution may have prevented another wave of death.

Cholera is deadly. It's also preventable and treatable. But around the world, millions died before doctors and scientists fully understood the disease and how it worked. Even with our knowledge, it still kills today.

KING CHOLERA

At first, the odds seem pretty good. Most people can withstand roughly a million cholera bacteria before getting sick. Then there's the bad news: This many microbes can hide in just a few ounces of water, and cholera bacteria are enthusiastic creatures. In only a few hours, they can reproduce into billions.

Cholera is gruesome and powerful. People used to call it "King Cholera" because of how it took control and ruled the body. It hits like a hammer and then works frighteningly fast. Some victims have died within two hours of getting sick!

The Blue Death

Cholera is caused by the bacterium known as *Vibrio cholerae*. These bacteria are endemic (naturally occurring) to the Ganges River in India. They thrive in warm, slightly salty water. They are also found in (or excreted in) human feces. In crowded, undeveloped areas, people's waste sometimes gets mixed in with their water supply. When people drink this polluted water, they drink the cholera bacteria, too. The bacteria can also live on the skins of fruits and vegetables.

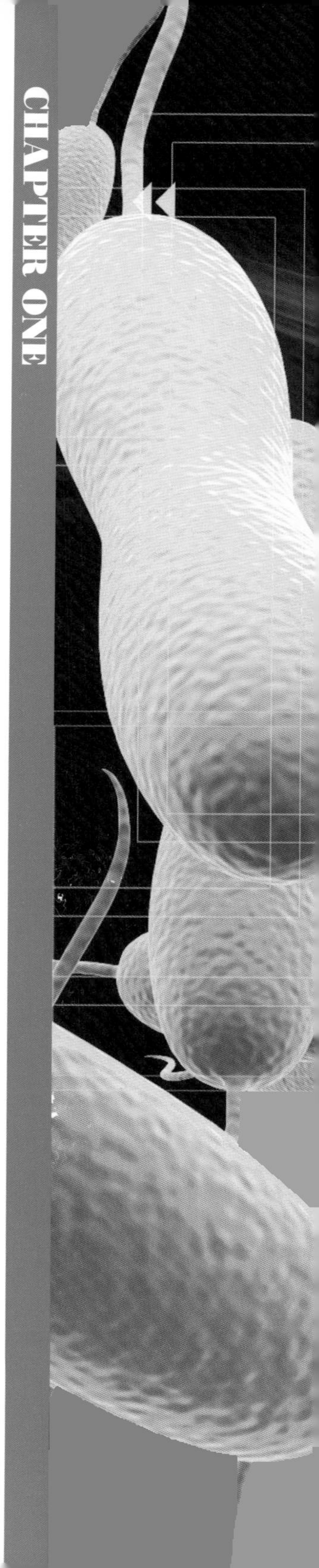

Once a person has cholera, he or she can easily give it to someone else. Vomiting and extreme diarrhea are the major symptoms of cholera. These fluids are full of cholera bacteria that can travel from person to person.

The stomach is a fighter—its powerful acids can kill the cholera bacterium. However, with so many bacteria swarming around, some of them escape down to the small intestine. The small intestine is more delicate. It can't kill the bacteria.

The cholera toxin works by interfering with cells in the body's small intestine. These cells are supposed to absorb water. Instead, cholera instructs them to purge water. This is what causes the diarrhea. It is watery and has a milky color, and it is often described as "rice-water."

People with cholera can lose quarts of water per day from diarrhea and vomiting. Some reports tell of victims who lose a third of their body weight, sometimes more, in just a few days. The exact origins of the word "cholera" are not known. Some experts think it comes from the Greek word for "gutter." Imagine the water gushing through a roof gutter after a rainstorm. That gives some idea of the violent diarrhea that strikes cholera victims.

Given enough time, cholera will work itself out of the body. Most victims don't have enough time, however. Death comes from something very basic: dehydration. As the body loses water, its cells desperately look around for more. They take water from the blood. As a result, the blood thickens and moves slowly. The heart can't pump enough blood through the body. (Patients have low blood volume, and their blood pressure drops.) The patient's pulse weakens. He or she may feel a tingling in the hands and feet. The eyes become sunken. The skin shrivels. The blood darkens, causing the person's skin to turn a dark blue. For this reason, cholera is sometimes called the blue death. Eventually, the victim loses

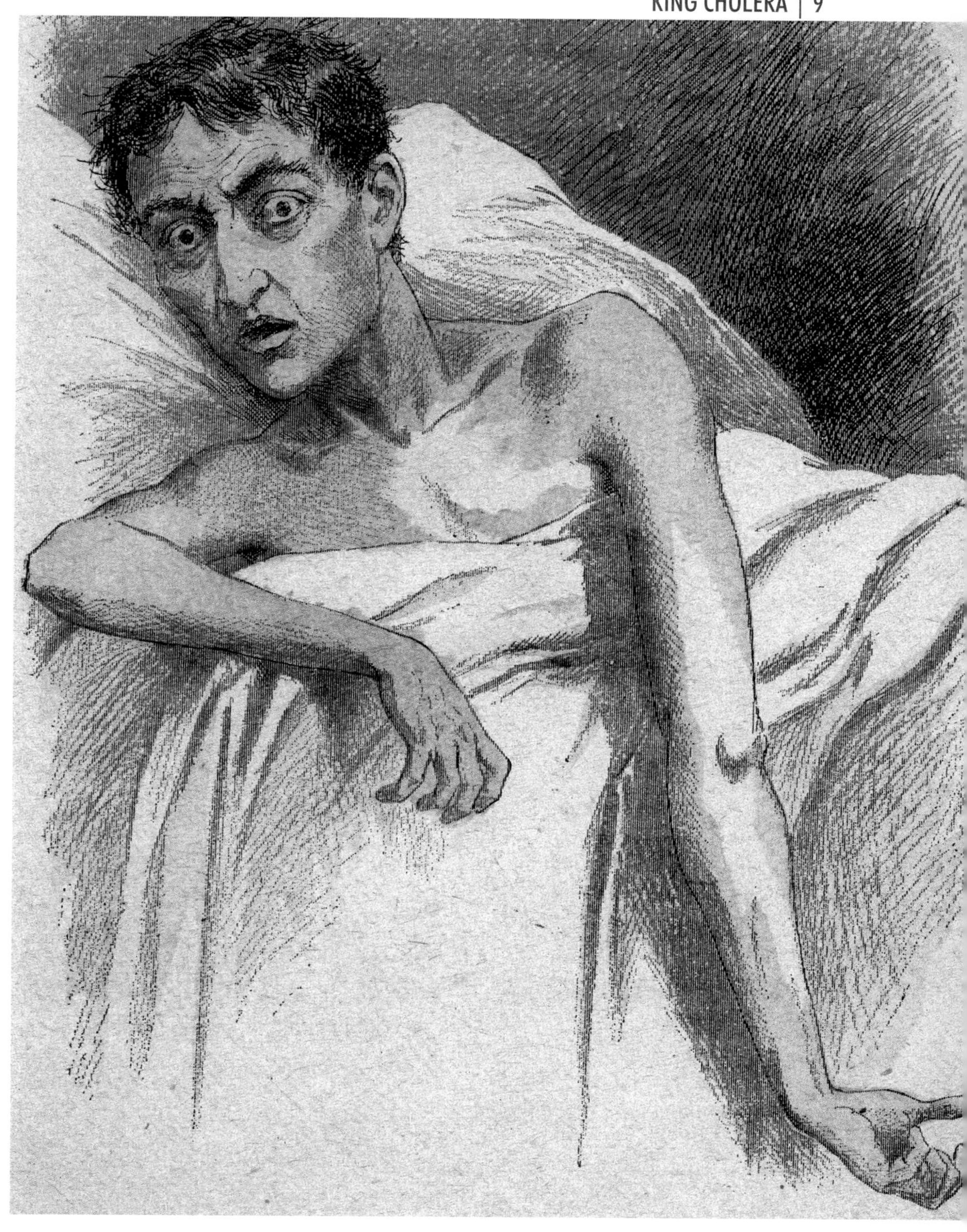

A cholera patient has a haunted look in this French medical book published in 1890. Sunken eyes were a common symptom of the disease.

consciousness—but that comes only at the very end. For most of this horrible process, the patient knows exactly what is happening. Within a few days, sometimes only a few hours, cholera kills about half of the people who get it.

Out of India

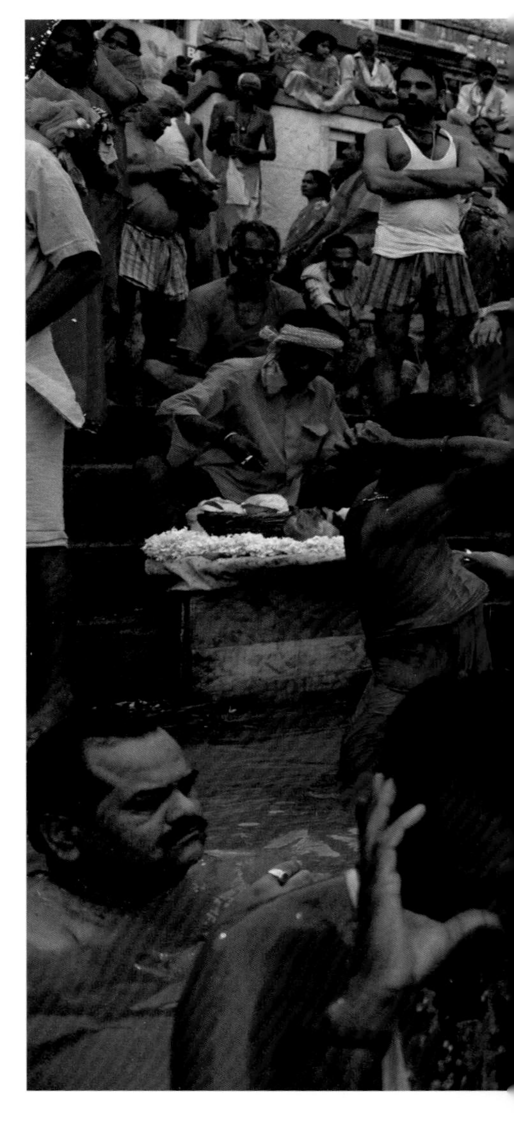

Cholera probably originated thousands of years ago. Ancient documents from about 500 BCE describe a disease that sounds like cholera. An outbreak in the late 1700s killed twenty thousand people in India. The disease also infected Europeans who had traveled to India. However, it had never left its home around the Ganges River.

The Ganges is an important part of India's main religion, Hinduism. Festivals and religious ceremonies are held there. In 1817, during a three-month-long festival, people used water from the river to drink and wash. Some of their waste flowed back into the river. Unfortunately, cholera bacteria were living in this waste. People got sick when they drank this infected water.

As Indians from all over the country traveled home, they took the disease with them. They contaminated their water back home. Hundreds of thousands of people died in Calcutta, India. Calcutta was an important port city. Sailors, soldiers, traders, and travelers moved through Calcutta every day on their way to somewhere else. Cholera had found a way out of

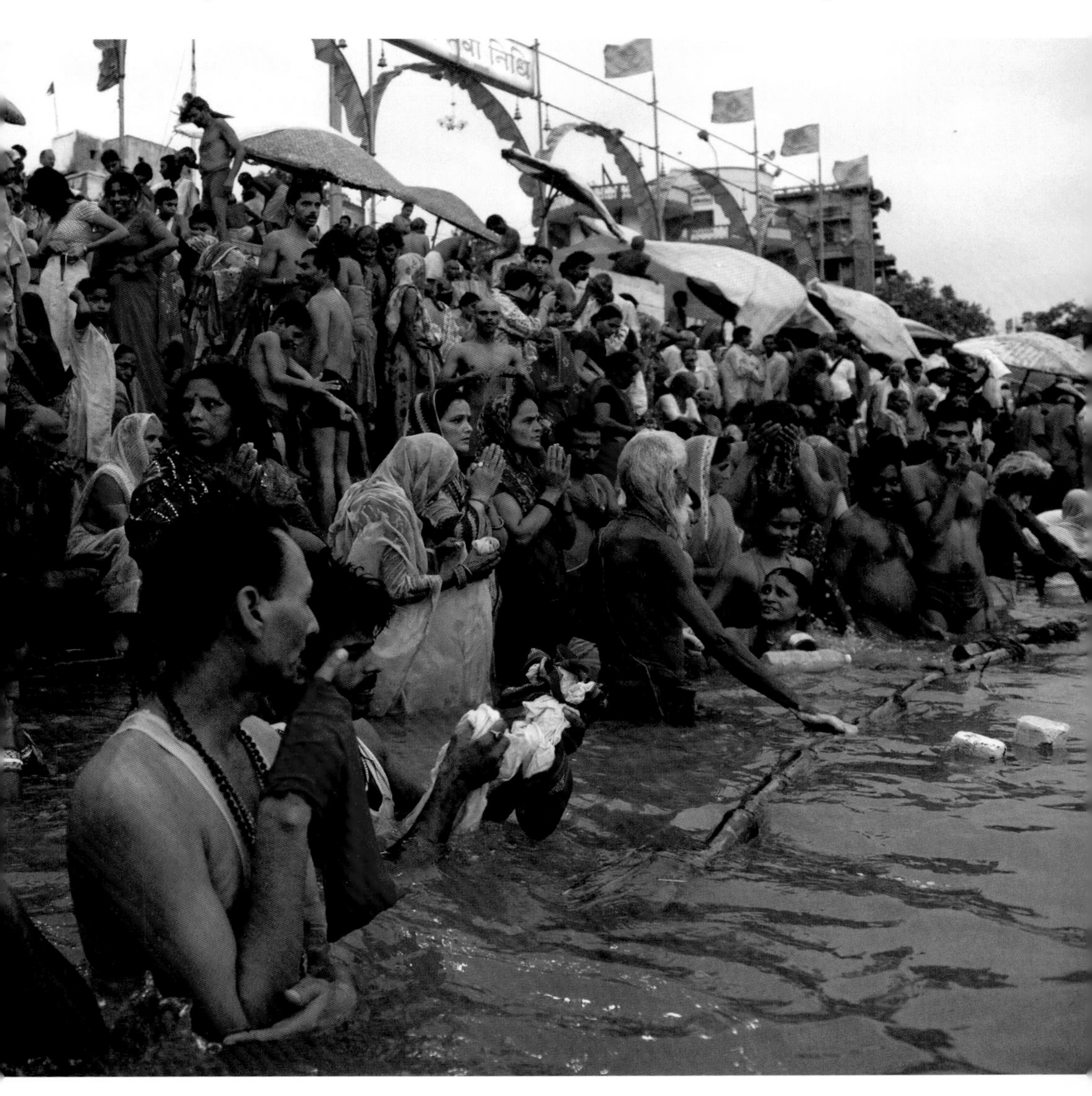

Hindu worshippers gather and bathe in India's Ganges River during a solar eclipse in 2009. The river plays an important part in India's main religion.

India. It traveled to Asia, Africa, and Russia. This was the start of the first pandemic (worldwide occurrence) of cholera. It would last until 1824.

Cities and Ships

Certain disease-causing microbes (pathogens) have always found humans to be good hosts. Microbes have one purpose in life: to spread. Humans offer microbes two attractive move-in bonuses. For one thing, we're social creatures. That makes it easy for microbes to spread from one person to another. And, whenever we can, we pack our bags and travel to new places. Bacteria can hitch a ride with us.

The Night Shift

People would have laughed at the idea of working nine to five in mid-nineteenth-century London. Vacation time? Forget it. Sick days? Nope. Societies were becoming more industrial. People used machines and worked in factories. They worked long hours, with few breaks, in conditions that were dirty, crowded, and often dangerous.

As bad as it was, there were probably not very many factory workers who wanted to trade places with workers in one of London's other professions: the night-rakers.

Working in the middle of the night, these men made the rounds of London's cesspools. They scooped out the human waste and loaded it into carts. Then they sold it to farmers who lived in the countryside near London. These farmers used it for fertilizer.

As London grew larger, it pushed outside of its original boundaries. Night-rakers had to travel even farther to sell their product, which made it more expensive. As a result, more and more of it was simply left to pile up. It either sat in the street or washed into the river, where it polluted precious drinking water.

In the 1800s, cities meant jobs. Things that had been made in people's houses were now produced in factories. People had to live near the factories where they worked. As a result, European cities became more and more crowded. People were jammed into rooms, which were jammed into buildings, which were jammed onto streets. Hundreds of people could live on 1 acre (0.4 hectare).

Some modern cities have populations this dense, too. But there's one major difference: plumbing.

Today, when you flush the toilet or scrape the remains of your dinner into the garbage disposal, that's the last you see of it. The waste flows into sewers. Sewers empty into a

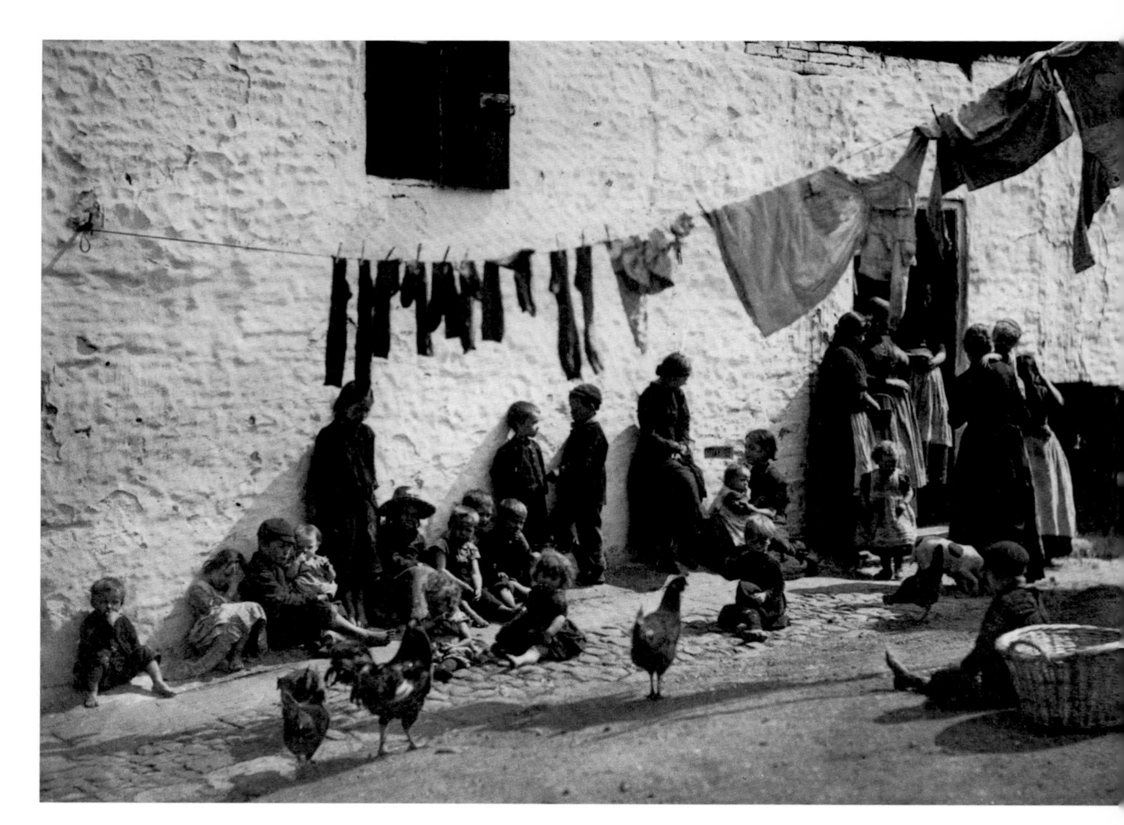

Children sit with animals and laundry outside a London slum in this 1889 photo. Cholera was a constant fear in crowded, dirty residences.

wastewater treatment plant. There, the waste is filtered out and the water is disinfected before being flushed out.

Things weren't so developed in the nineteenth century, however. Take London as an example. Waste was dumped into the gutter. When it rained, the water carried everything straight into the Thames River.

When people needed water, they got it from various pumps throughout the city. From where did the pumps draw water? The Thames River! The same waste that people had just tried to get rid of was on its way back.

Also throughout the nineteenth century, travel was getting faster, easier, and more common. International shipping was a booming business. Railroads were being laid across Europe and the United States. These new travel routes made getting around much easier for people—and made it easier to spread the disease-causing microbes they carried.

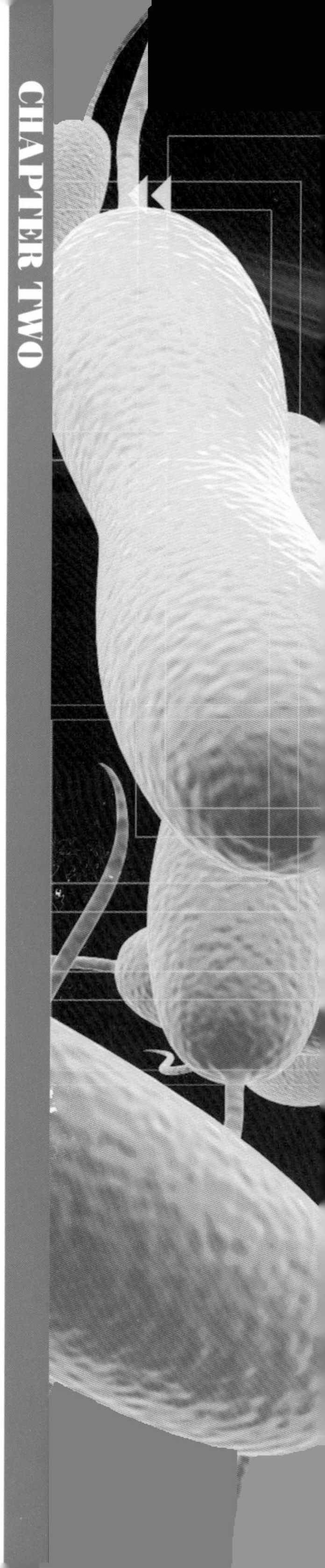

A GLOBAL PROBLEM

In the last two hundred years, the world has experienced seven cholera pandemics. A pandemic is a major outbreak that affects many people and spreads over a large area. For centuries, cholera stayed in India. But by the beginning of the nineteenth century, human progress had turned it into a worldwide disease.

Moving North

The first pandemic lasted from about 1817 to 1824. In 1827, cholera left India again. The disease preferred warm weather. Nevertheless, it made its way into the chilly regions of Russia and Europe.

The city of Astrakhan, about 900 miles (1,448 kilometers) from Moscow, was ravaged. The bank closed. The marketplace was deserted. Bodies lay in the streets where they had fallen. Gravediggers were overwhelmed by the task facing them. They dug a pit and threw a thousand corpses into it.

Cholera headed north, to Moscow. By November 1830, five thousand of Moscow's citizens had fallen ill. More than half died. Next the

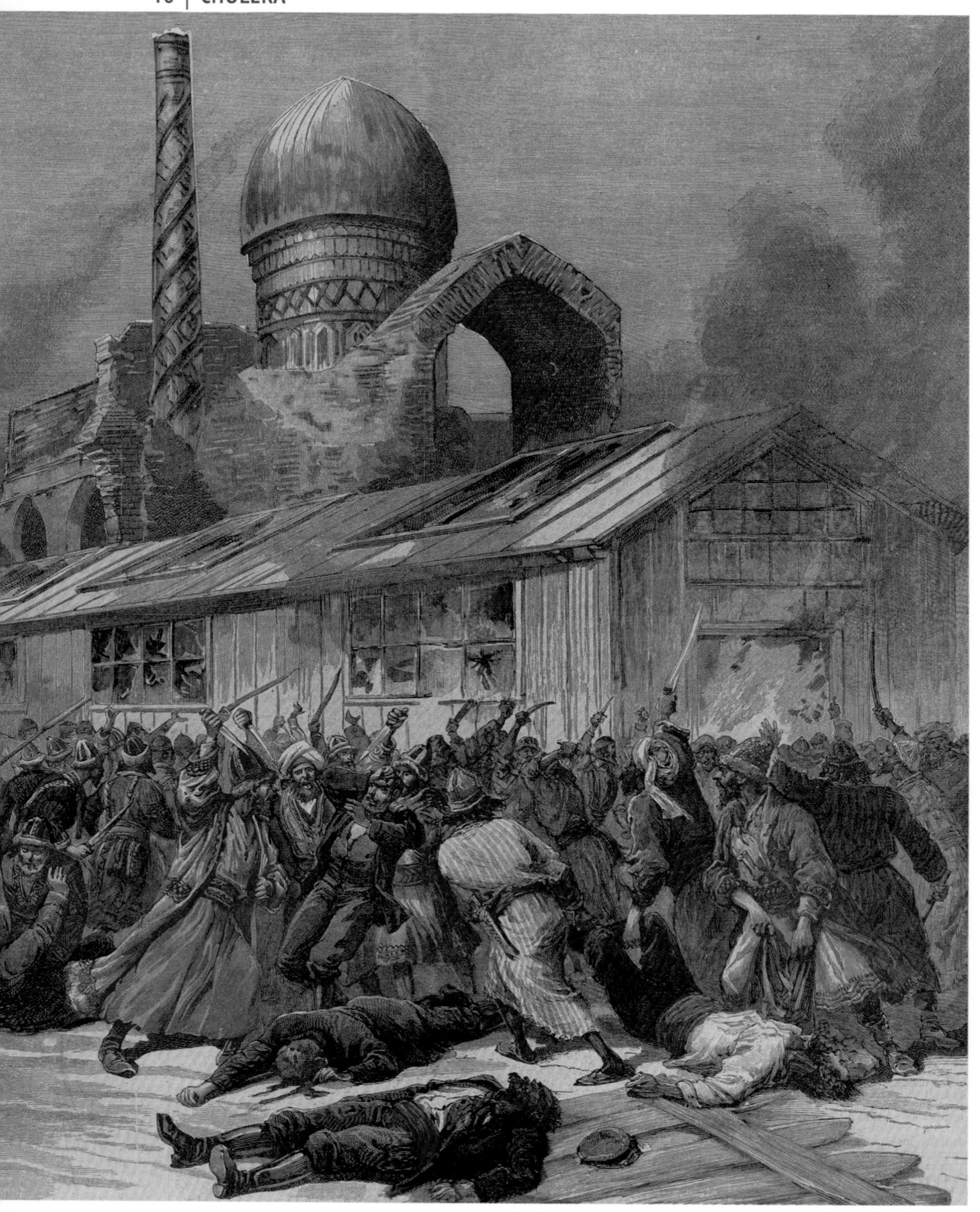

People rioted as cholera spread through Russia in the 1830s. An artist's interpretation is shown here in an 1892 drawing called *The Troubles in Astrakhan*.

disease moved into St. Petersburg. By the summer of 1831, the city's population had been cut down by ten thousand.

Russian officials were worried. They held an essay contest, offering a big prize to anyone who could explain the horrid disease. What was it? Where did it come from? Most important, how could it be stopped? But there was no stopping cholera.

The English were worried, too. They knew cholera spread quickly and killed easily. England wasn't safe. Its many port towns welcomed ships from all over the world, including Russia. It seemed to be only a matter of time before one of them brought cholera.

Officials tried to protect the country. They quarantined any incoming ships from Russia, where cholera had claimed so many lives. But cholera was a disease that slipped through the water effortlessly. It found a way in.

William Sproat was a river man from a town called Sunderland. He was England's first recorded case of cholera. (Records now show there were earlier victims; however, the cause of their deaths was not recognized at the time.) Sproat passed the disease to his family. Then it spread through the town. Sunderland was placed under quarantine for a week. Movement in and out of the town was severely limited or prohibited. Quarantines were good health policy: they could help slow down the spread of disease. However, they were disastrous for the economy. Sunderland was a small port town. Its residents made their living by the trading ships that came to its docks. People suffered when the docks remained empty. After a week, doctors reported that cholera was not in Sunderland after all! This false announcement gave cholera permission to spread even farther. It moved down the coast. Finally, it reached London. It killed thousands before winter arrived and cold weather stopped it.

During this outbreak (1831–1832), a young English doctor named John Snow saw his first cholera victims. Like other doctors of his time, Snow did not know how to help people who had it. But he was curious about the strange disease, and when cholera returned in later years, Snow was there to study it.

Across the Atlantic

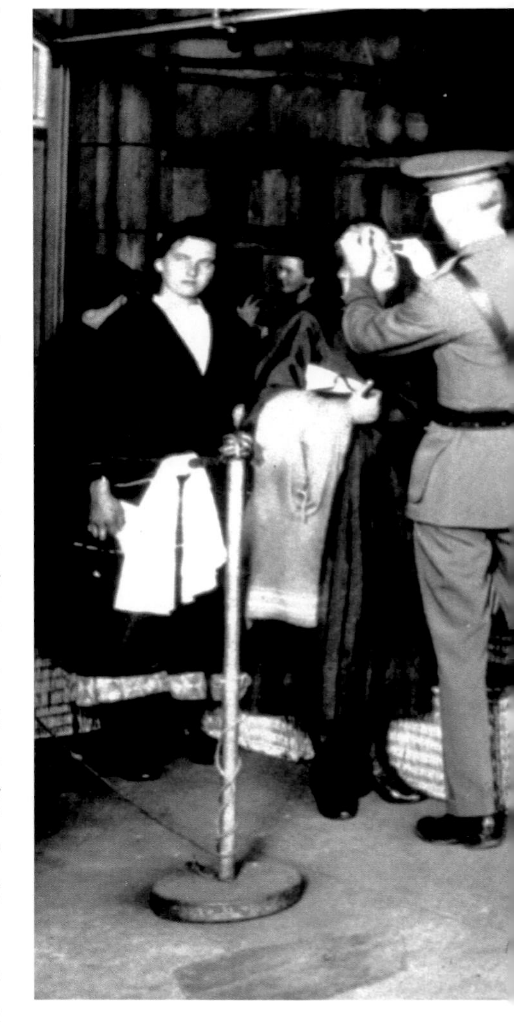

Cholera paid no attention to national boundaries. It hit Russia and Great Britain. Then it moved through the rest of Europe, including the Mediterranean, as well as Asia and Africa.

In 1832, British ships loaded up a deadly export. Immigrants—most of them Irish—were looking for a better life in the Americas. They piled into ships for the journey across the Atlantic Ocean. Many of these people were desperately poor and literally starving. They had few possessions. But they did bring one thing: cholera. In the cramped quarters of ships, the disease spread rapidly. Many people died during the trip. Many more arrived sick.

Ships from England were quarantined. But this did not stop the disease—or desperate immigrants. In the summer of 1832, more than fifty thousand immigrants arrived in Canada.

Cholera broke out in Montreal. It quickly moved south as immigrants made their way to the United States. The disease hit a few places in upstate New York, gathering strength as it headed for its next stop: New York City.

If cholera reached a large, populated city, it would be nearly impossible to stop. Word traveled quickly around the

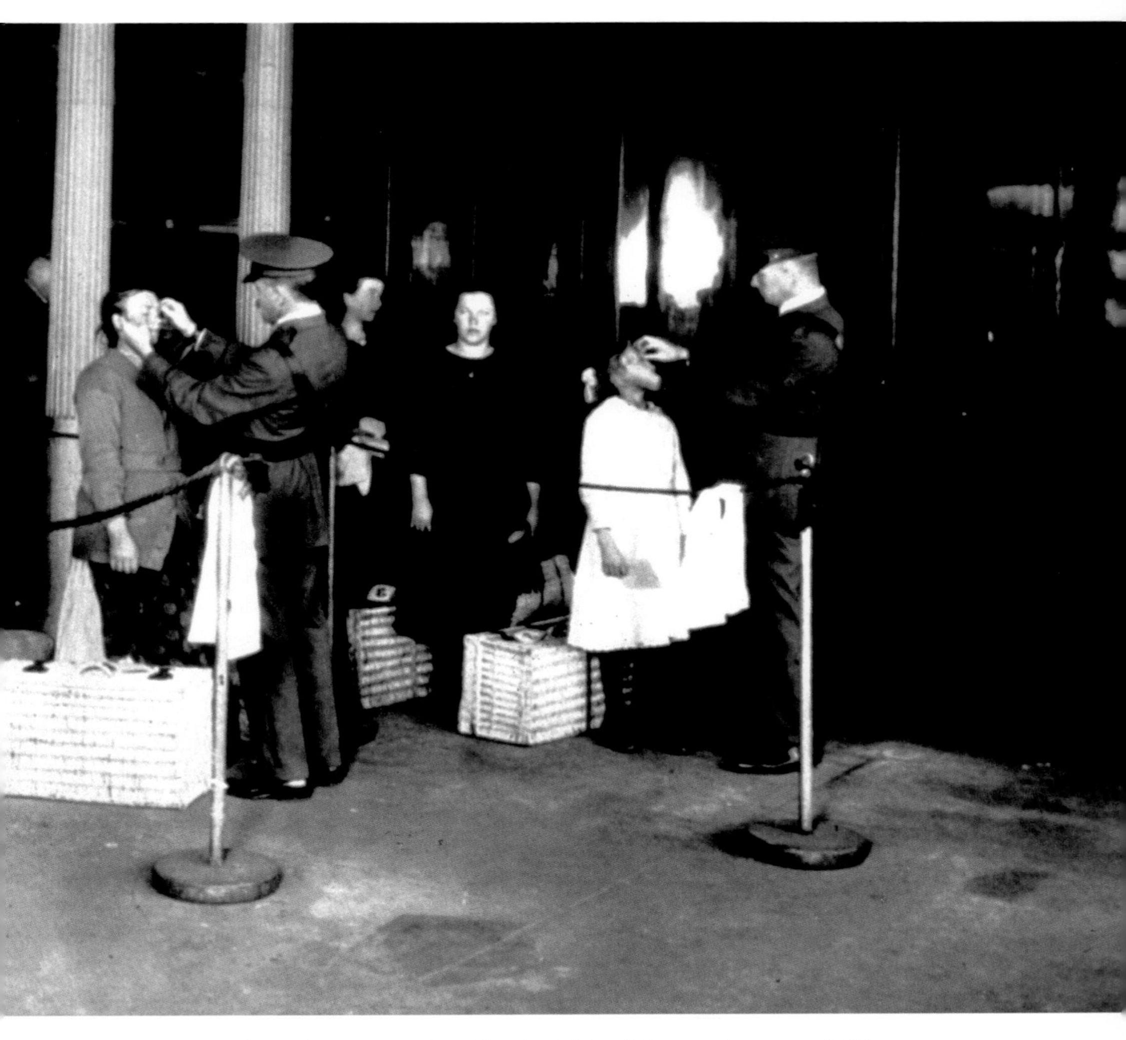

Thousands of immigrants arrived in the United States by way of Ellis Island in New York. Before they were allowed to enter the country, they were checked for signs of disease.

city. Residents began fleeing. They could not all escape, however. By August, cholera had killed about 3,500 New Yorkers.

After cholera invaded New York, it continued to spread across the United States—to Boston, Philadelphia, Chicago, and St. Louis. Some cities were hit worse than others. New Orleans, being in a warm climate with so much water, was an ideal home for cholera. In the fall of 1832, New Orleans lost five thousand residents.

Cholera Returns

In 1831 and 1832, cholera made its way through Europe, Russia, and the United States in a matter of months. And then it vanished—for fifteen years.

President Jackson's Decision

In the 1830s, religion was an important part of life in America. In 1832, Christian churches across the country led their congregations in days of fasting and prayer. Many Christians thought God sent diseases such as cholera as punishment for sin. To get rid of disease, they thought they needed to behave in ways that were morally correct and show regret for past sins. They hoped such appeals to God would protect them from, or at least lessen, the disease.

President Andrew Jackson was asked to recommend a national day of fasting. Although he was quick to say that he believed in the power of prayer, he refused to declare a national day of fasting. Jackson said this would go against the Constitution, which established the rights of U.S. citizens. The Constitution said that matters of church and state (government) should be kept separate. Jackson was strongly criticized for his position. Some believed his decision showed how Americans did not honor God, which was the reason they had gotten cholera in the first place.

When it returned, the cholera bacterium was ready for new victims. Just as before, the disease began in India. It moved through the Middle East and into the Mediterranean. It then spread into Europe and Africa. Cholera killed thousands everywhere it went.

Again it crossed the Atlantic. A famine in Ireland had sent a new wave of immigrants to North America. However, cholera and other diseases broke out on the ships. In the spring and summer of 1847, hundreds of ships arrived at the Canadian port of Grosse Île. Sick people poured off the boats, and thousands died.

As it had fifteen years earlier, cholera filtered down to New York and across the United States. This epidemic coincided with another huge event in American history. In 1848 and 1849, thousands of people were moving west on what was called the Oregon Trail. Some of them were hoping to make their fortunes by mining gold that had been found in Oregon and California. Others just wanted to set up a homestead in the unsettled lands of the West.

Many of these pioneers never made it. They came down with cholera. Living in close quarters, they easily passed it to each other. The trail across the United States was studded with graves. Piles of stones were topped with a simple wooden cross marked with the person's name and the word "cholera."

In 1852, the third pandemic of cholera began. By now, scientists were seriously studying the disease. If they could figure out what caused it, perhaps they could also figure out how to stop it. In 1854, during the Broad Street outbreak in London, John Snow's research proved vital to understanding—and eventually stopping—the disease. However, the importance of his discoveries would not be recognized until years later.

Cholera was far from conquered. The third pandemic lasted until about 1860. There was only a short break before the fourth pandemic occurred from 1863 to 1879. The fifth raged from 1881 to 1896, and the sixth began in 1899 and lasted until 1923. Although doctors and scientists were beginning to understand the disease, it was still too powerful to stop.

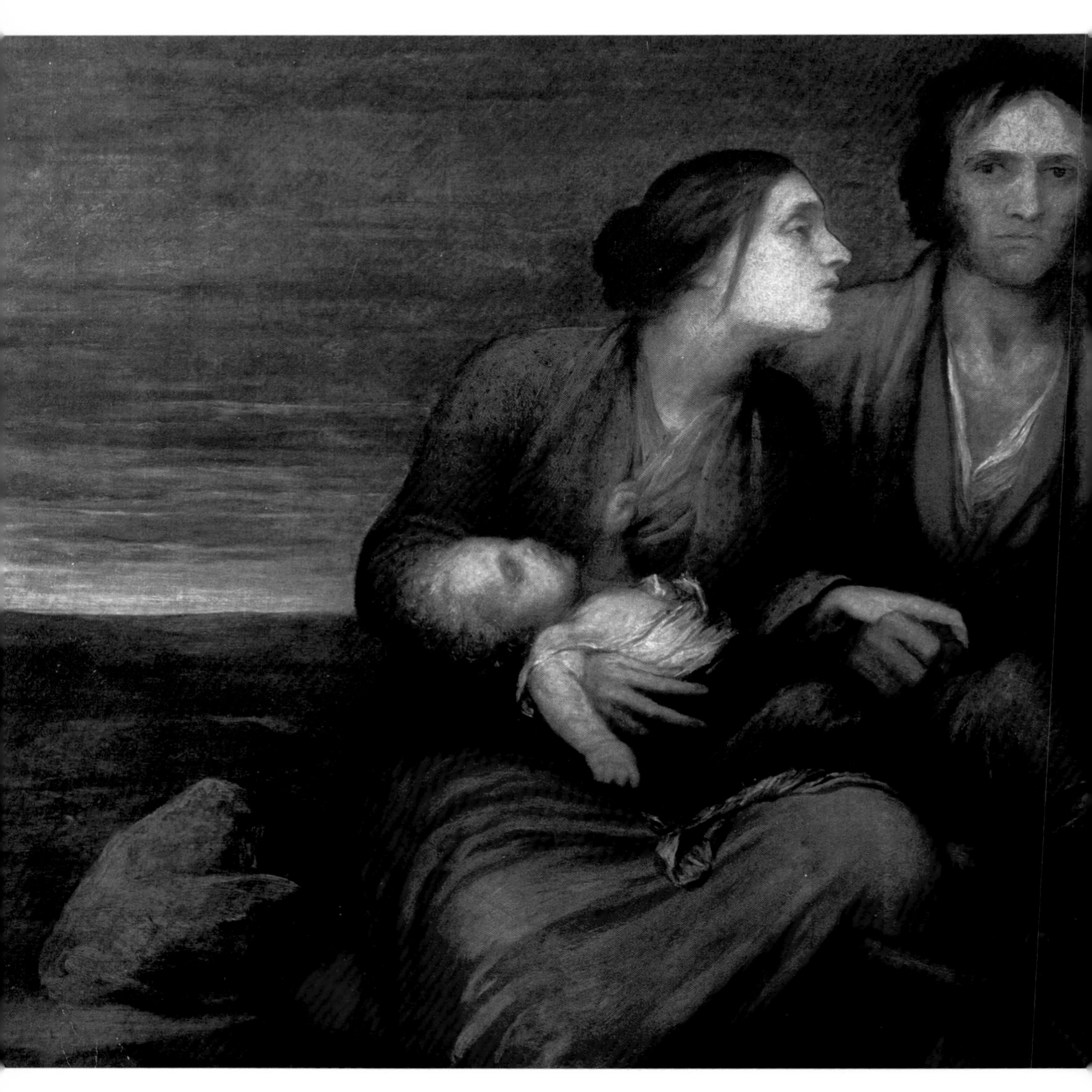

This oil painting by George Frederick Watts shows a desperate family during the Irish famine of the mid-1800s. The food shortage drove many starving people to immigrate to the Americas.

The seventh pandemic began in 1961, with a new strain of the cholera bacterium. Another new strain was discovered in 1992.

Cholera remains a global problem. Developing countries are more affected because they often do not have reliable sources of clean water. However, developed regions, such as the United States and most of Europe, still get isolated cases. Many of these cases happen when citizens travel to undeveloped countries, where they pick up the disease and then bring it home with them. Fortunately, cholera can be stopped quickly with good medical care.

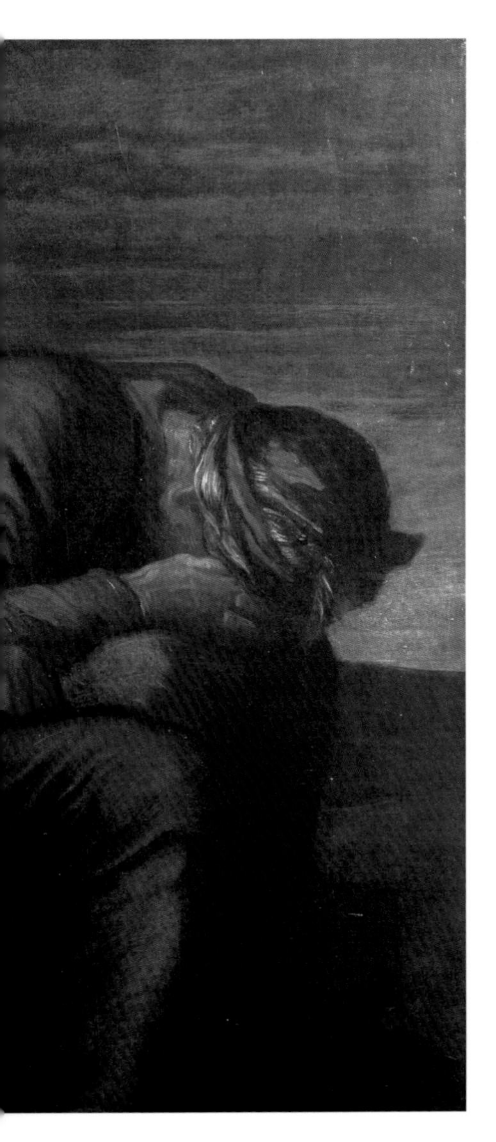

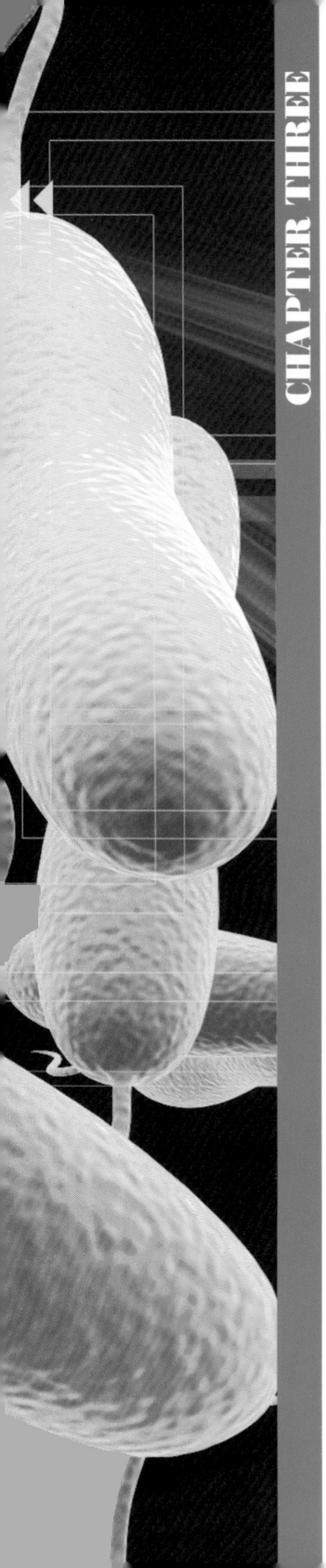

THE LIVING DEATH

In the nineteenth century, there were few things worse than having cholera "in the house." People were shunned by their neighbors and friends. Even members of their own family might shut them out. A man in England lost his wife and two sons to the disease. Neighbors blamed him for bringing the disease to the community. Some people fled their homes to avoid angry neighbors. Others—too sick or too poor to run—were simply abandoned. They had to fend for themselves the best they could.

Remedies

Medicine in the nineteenth century still relied on old theories. Nobody knew what caused cholera. Doctors didn't even know how to treat its most obvious and dangerous symptom—diarrhea.

As cholera victims became dehydrated, their blood became thicker. This made many doctors think that cholera was, in fact, a blood disease. They believed the solution was to "bleed" the patient. They literally opened a patient's veins and let the blood run out. They believed this would rid the body of the toxin.

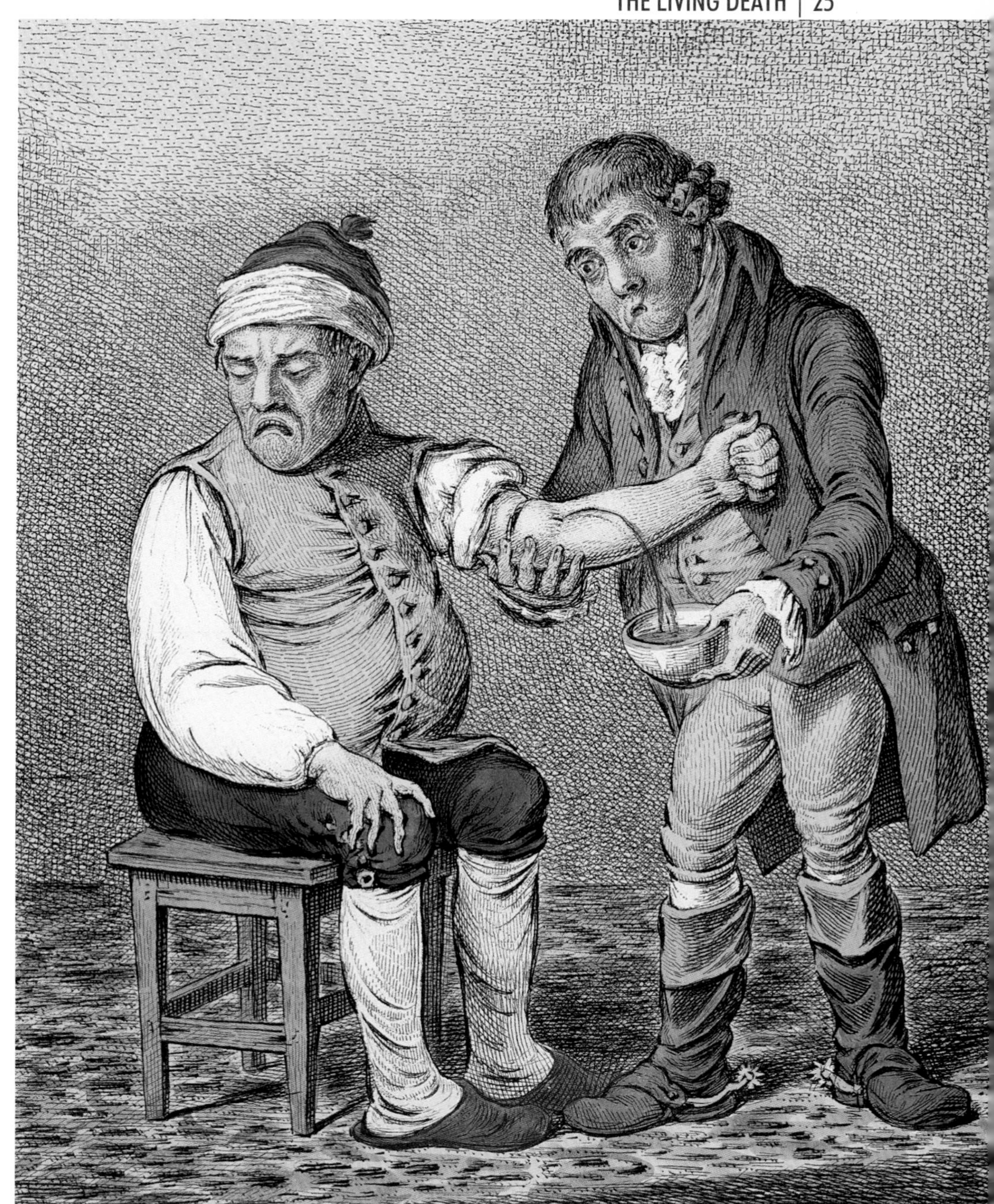

Bloodletting was an accepted medical practice in the 1900s. Many doctors believed that cholera was a blood disease and that the best way to treat it was to bleed out the poison.

Doctors also thought that vomiting and diarrhea were the body's ways of trying to get rid of poisons. They often prescribed medicines that would increase these symptoms. This was the worst thing they could have done. Patients who were already severely dehydrated were losing more of their vital fluids.

Camphor, which comes from a certain evergreen tree, was a popular remedy. However, this treatment caused vomiting, not to mention dizziness and muscle spasms. Sometimes it even caused respiratory failure (not being able to breathe). Calomel was also widely used, but this drug was no better. It was a type of mercury, which is extremely poisonous and can be fatal.

Herbal remedies were everywhere. There were mint and mustard, vinegar and wine. All kinds of household items were

A Deadly Christmas Present

Three days after Christmas in 1832, an English man named John Barnes became sick with cholera and died. His wife and two other people also became ill (although they recovered). Then three more people got sick.

It was clear Barnes had infected those around him. But how had he gotten sick? Doctors were stumped. Then Barnes's son arrived in town. He reported that his aunt, John Barnes's sister, had died from cholera two weeks before. Her clothes had been sent back to the Barnes family. They had not been washed. On Christmas Day, John Barnes opened the package and freed the deadly cholera bacterium.

After Barnes's wife got sick, her mother came to help care for her. She nursed her daughter back to health, but she collapsed on her way back home. She then gave the disease to her husband and another daughter. All three died.

Barnes lost her husband, her parents, and her sister within the course of about a week—all because of a package of used clothing.

sniffed, swallowed, or applied to the skin. One doctor ordered that toast be soaked in vinegar, sprinkled with pepper, and then laid on the victim's abdomen. Another doctor recommended that a moist compact of bran be pressed between sheets and wrapped around the patient's legs. Burning tar to purify the air was considered helpful. So was meat smothered in garlic. Electric shock therapy? Leeches? Ice baths? All were tried. The one thing that could have helped—water—was rarely suggested.

Fear of Doctors

Many people did not trust the care offered by doctors or local authorities. It usually didn't help, and it often made things worse. They were better off trying to take care of themselves, using simple solutions like eating chicken soup—which was far more helpful.

If getting a doctor's care was risky, going to the hospital was considered a death sentence. In fact, people who entered hospitals did die at alarming rates. That was partly because only very sick patients—those likely to die anyway—went to the hospital in the first place. Still, the hospital was avoided at all costs. People would deny they had sick family members, or they would try to hide them—anything to keep them home. A doctor in Paris, France, told the story of an elderly couple, sick with cholera, who had nowhere to sleep. When he suggested the hospital, they refused. They said they "preferred to die."

People were also afraid that doctors would declare someone dead before he or she really was. Cholera was called the living death because its victims looked dead, even when they were not. The blood doesn't circulate well and, as a result, the skin turns blue. The eyes become unfocused. The pulse becomes so weak that it might not be felt. Without oxygen

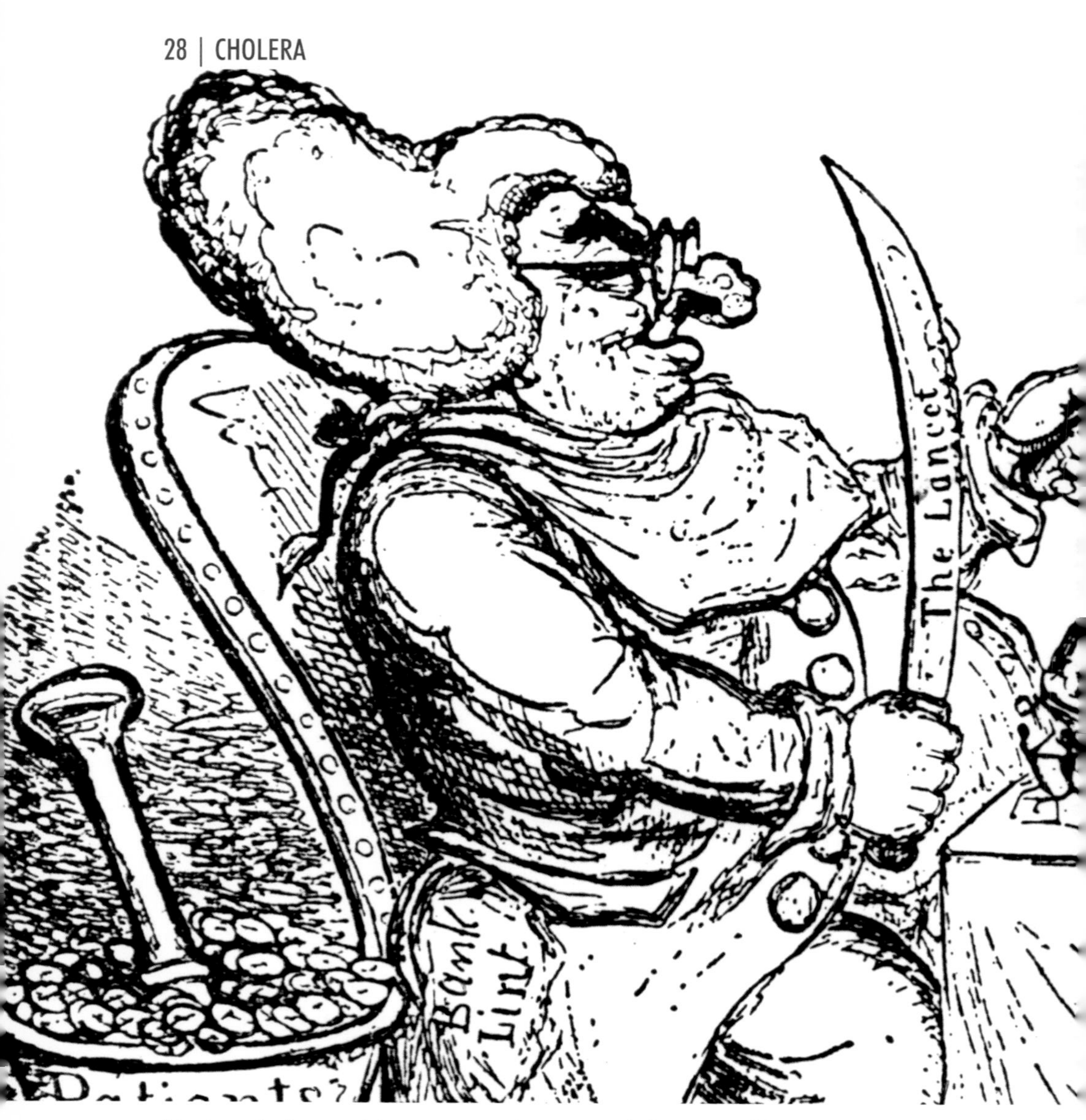

During cholera epidemics, people accused doctors of being greedy and collecting money even when they could not offer any help. This cartoon shows a doctor getting rich off the disease.

reaching the brain, the patient sinks into a coma. He or she looks dead. In 1832, one doctor reported, "It is so easy to be completely mistaken that I once marked down as dead an individual who in fact died several hours later."

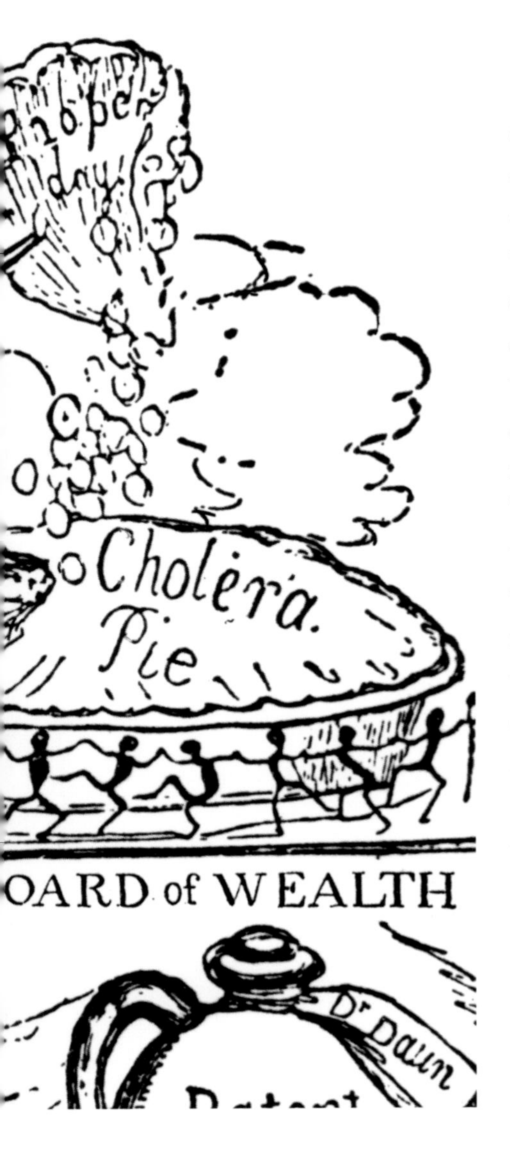

The fear of being buried alive was horrible—and not entirely unfounded. There was often a rush to bury cholera victims before they infected other people. When people did die, their relatives tried to protect their bodies. Some were afraid that the victims would not receive a proper burial. They also feared that doctors would use their corpses to practice dissection. In the nineteenth century, doctors were desperate for bodies they could study. To learn more about the human body, they needed to do autopsies. Legally, they could only use the bodies of criminals, but there were only so many dead criminals to go around. Grave robbing was a thriving, if illegal, business. People would literally take bodies out of their graves and sell them to doctors who wanted to dissect them.

It was difficult to keep track of a body during an epidemic. Officials sometimes took corpses forcibly and buried them in special graves for cholera victims. However, people often feared their loved ones were really ending up in the hands of greedy doctors.

In one New York apartment building, people tried to stop the authorities from removing a body. The authorities finally had to lower the coffin out of the window.

Problems for Survivors

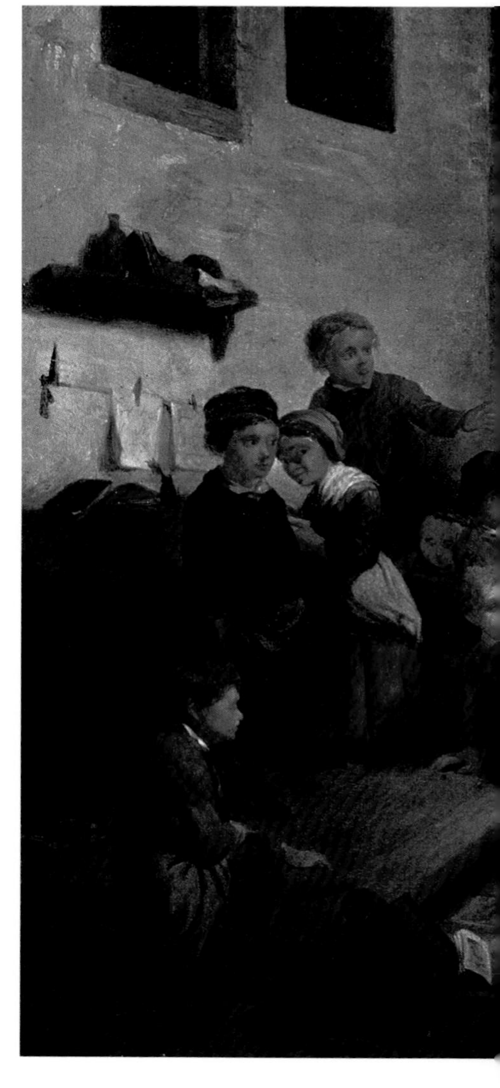

Children today are vaccinated against killer diseases. But in the nineteenth century, disease was simply a part of life. It sounds coldhearted, but parents usually expected some of their children to die. However, by the time people reached adulthood, most of them were safe.

Cholera affected families a little differently. It killed adults. Adults in a family did most of the work—bringing in money or taking care of children or elderly relatives. Their deaths were devastating, especially for poor people who had no money or support system. In England, for example, widows and orphans might fall under the Poor Law. This was a crude, harsh welfare system for people who could not support themselves. Under this law, people lived in special quarters and had almost no privileges. Families were split up. Orphanages were often bleak, depressing places. Children could be underfed, overworked, and abused.

As if the loss of a family member wasn't bad enough, families suffered financial losses as well. According to the law,

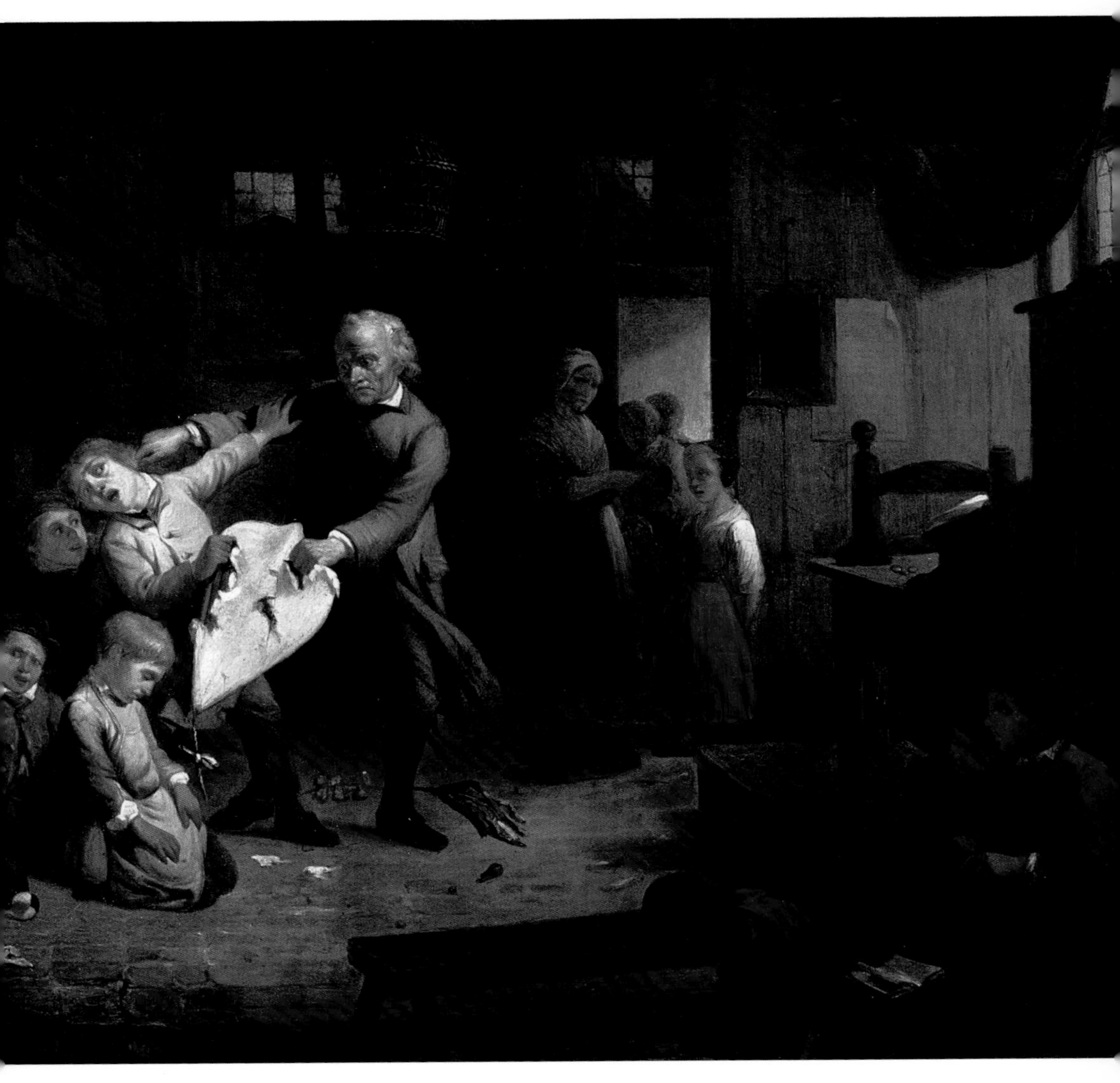

A child is punished while his peers look on in this nineteenth-century painting. Poor children who lost their parents to cholera might end up in orphanages where they were mistreated.

a cholera victim's personal belongings had to be burned. This was a health policy intended to stop the disease from spreading. However, it created a hardship for poor families. They had no clothing, bedding, or dishes to spare. Some people asked their local governments to pay them back for the cost of the destroyed items. These requests were sometimes granted.

Affluent people suffered different kinds of losses. In cities, people abandoned their houses when they fled, leaving their properties open to vandalism or theft. Staying put came with another set of problems. Merchants struggled to find customers. Customers struggled to find basic supplies. In 1832, one New York woman wrote that she could not even buy a loaf of bread.

When cholera hit, posters and notices were tacked up all over town, announcing the disease's arrival. In only a few weeks, cholera could shut down a city. New York, Paris, London, and Moscow were places where business and culture had thrived. But during a cholera epidemic, only one thing mattered: staying alive.

Myths and Facts

MYTH You will catch cholera if you come into contact with someone who has it.

FACT While cholera is highly contagious, the immune and digestive systems have the ability to fight back, sometimes before the disease has the chance to spread throughout the body. If you are traveling in a country where cholera cases have recently occurred, wash your hands frequently and be careful to avoid food and beverages that have not been carefully washed in or made with clean water.

MYTH People get cholera because they aren't clean.

FACT Cholera can spread in many different ways and to people who are very careful about cleanliness. It can spread through the water and personal contact with people who are sick.

MYTH Cholera has been completely eradicated.

FACT Cases of cholera still occur occasionally around the world. But now that doctors are better equipped to deal with it, the number of deaths and infections has drastically gone down.

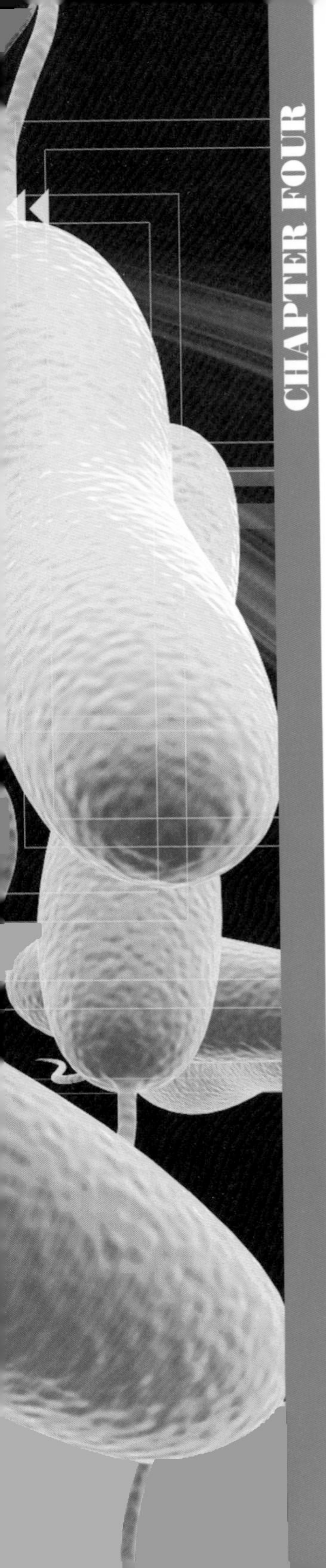

A SOCIAL CRISIS

Nobody knew what caused cholera or how to stop it. Most people recognized that squalid conditions and disease were connected. However, they did not realize the link was the cholera bacterium. Instead, they believed that miasmas—polluted air caused by bad smells—were at fault. They also thought disease was more likely to strike people with low moral standards.

The evidence for what caused cholera was there, but it would take years for doctors and scientists to piece it together. Until then, fear, suspicion, and flat-out panic drove people to violence or into hiding.

Desperate Measures

Although nineteenth-century people felt powerless to do anything about cholera, it wasn't for lack of trying. Doctors offered what little knowledge they had. Officials organized cleanup efforts. They required citizens to clean up outside their own homes. Extra men were hired to remove garbage and waste from the streets. Organizations of nurses and volunteers tried to care for the poor and the sick.

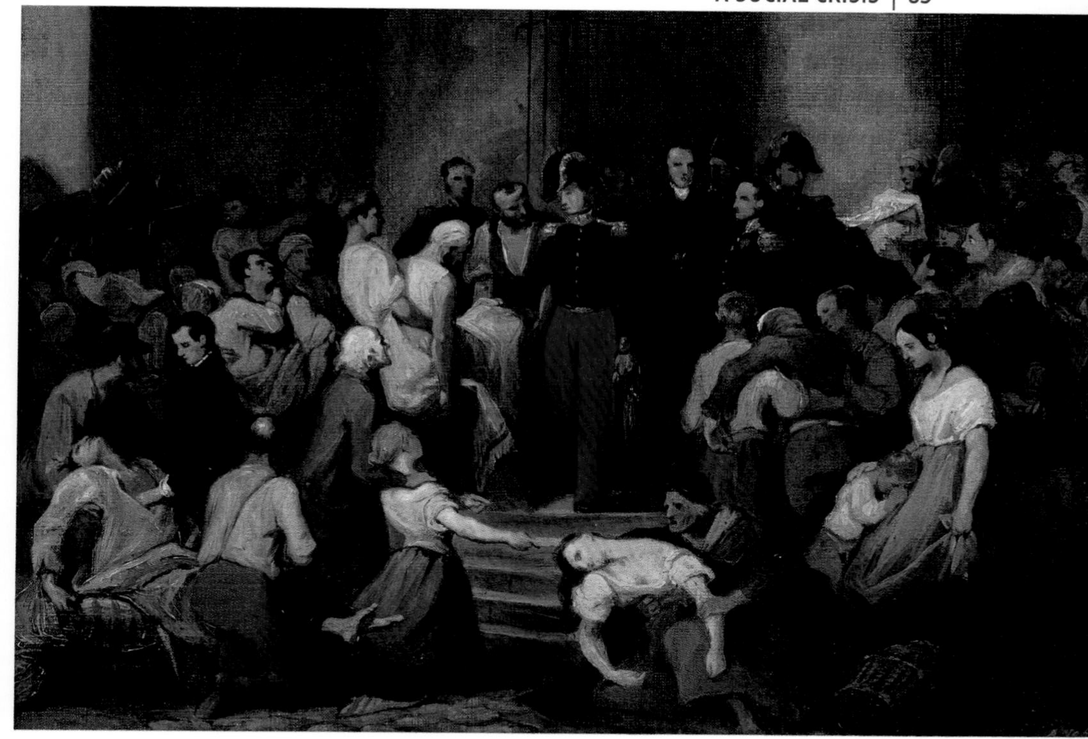

Cholera patients were treated at l'Hôtel-Dieu, a hospital in Paris, during the 1832 epidemic. In this painting, a member of the nobility, the Duke of Orléans, visits the sick. Many of those ill were of the lower classes.

Some efforts backfired. On a practical level, cleaning up during an epidemic was risky. It was just as likely to spread the disease as it was to eliminate it. Moving people to hospitals only exposed more to the disease. Those who did make it to the hospital were not ensured good care, anyway. And charity was often insulting to the people who received it.

In 1849, some New Yorkers tried to convert schools into temporary hospitals. However, some people worried that after the buildings had been used as cholera hospitals, no one would want to use them as schools. Also, they would be turning out the students who attended them. With nothing to do, the children might pick up bad habits, and that would make them more susceptible to the disease.

Dealing with the dead was a huge problem. At the height of an epidemic, hundreds of people could die in a single day. Coffin makers could not keep up. Also, it was difficult to find people willing to handle the corpses. They were afraid of being infected. Sometimes the corpses were collected on carts. Other times, they just piled up in the streets. The ritual of the funeral soon fell by the wayside. People were so busy trying to stay alive that they had nothing left for the dead.

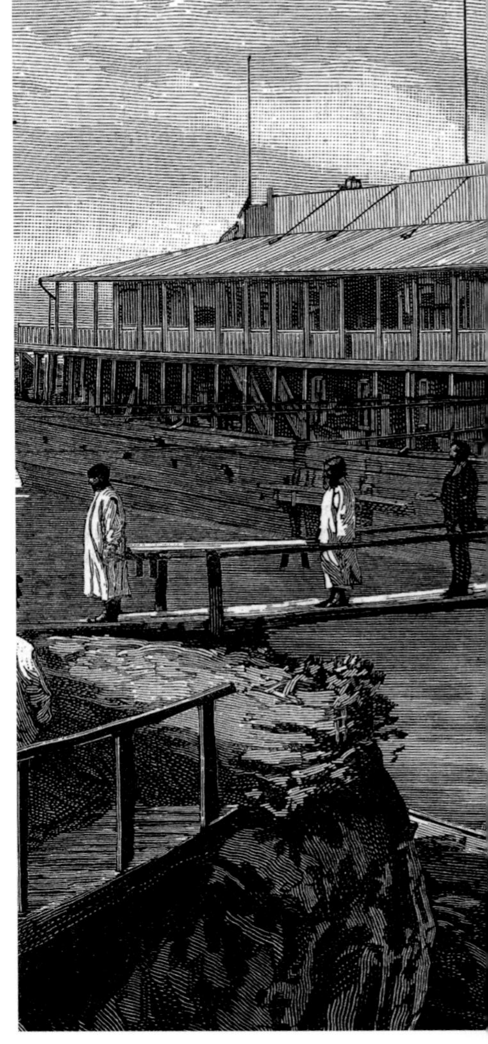

Social Unrest

In the 1800s, medicine underwent a revolution. At the beginning of the century, many doctors still relied on scientific theories that had been formed hundreds of years before. However, by the end of the century, there would be breakthroughs in anesthesia and surgery. There would be new theories about disease-causing microbes and new approaches about how to diagnose patients infected by them.

Cholera fell right in the middle of this change. As old thought met new, doctors disagreed with one another. Adding to the problem was that anyone could call himself a doctor. He needed no education, no training, and no license. Mostly, he just had to act convincing enough to attract customers. Not all doctors were frauds, of course, but there were no consistent standards.

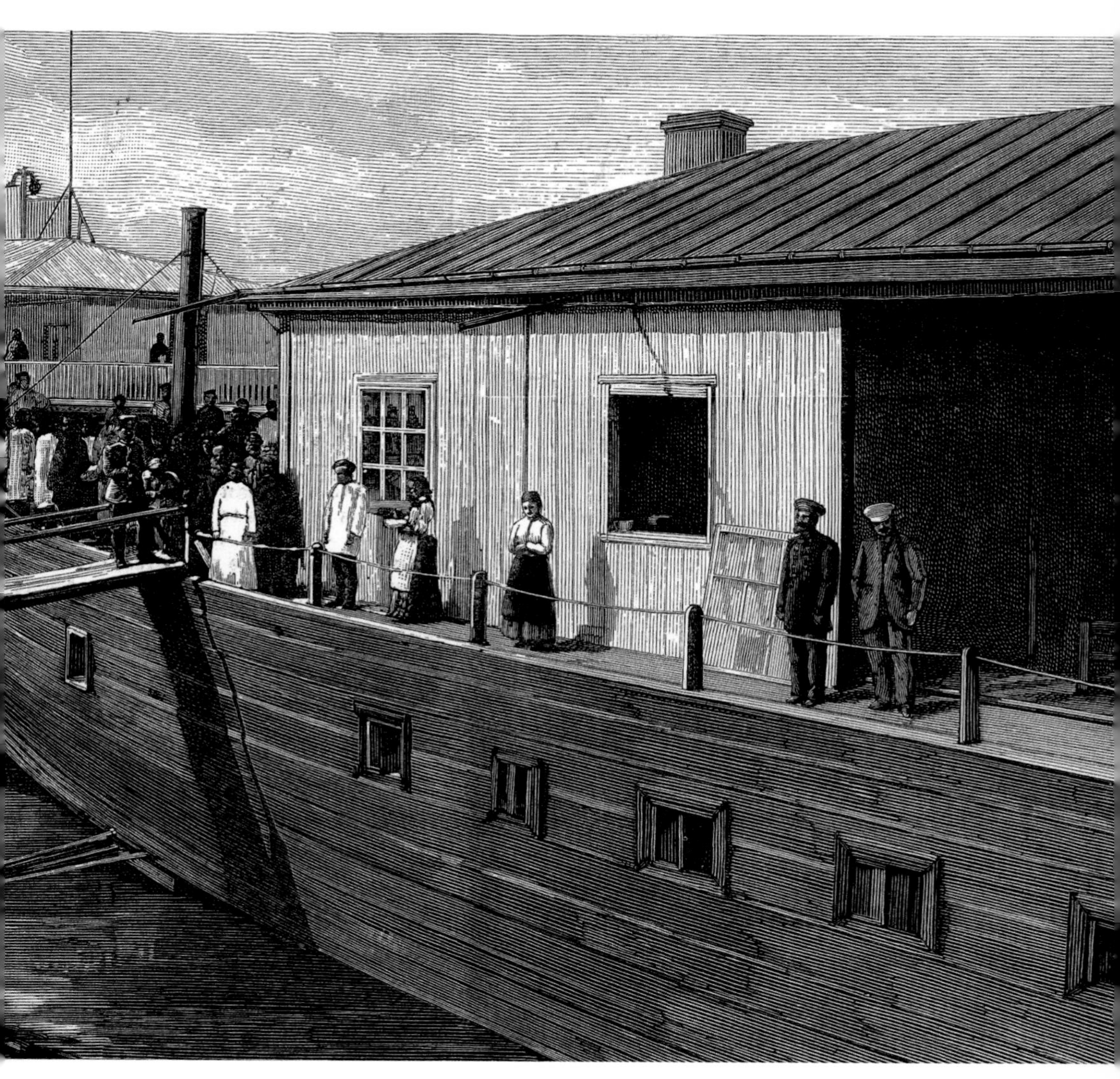

During cholera epidemics, such as the one in Russia pictured here, ships were quarantined and refused entry into ports. Many people were stranded on board.

The failure to find answers or provide reliable care made people angry and fearful. Terrified people looked for a cause, a pattern, a source—anything that they could blame. All over the world, frightened and angry people attacked doctors, the nobility, and other authorities. Panic spread through the streets faster than the disease itself.

Throughout England, crowds attacked hospitals. They broke the windows, destroyed beds and furniture, and freed the sick. A doctor in Paris wrote in his memoir that he was "threatened, insulted, [and] treated as a poisoner." He described a riot in front of a local hospital. "If at that moment someone had revealed my profession, I would have been torn to pieces," he wrote.

In Russia, the police rounded up sick people and forced them to go to hospitals. There, the patients' clothes were taken and they were given drugs to halt the disease. They were beaten if they tried to resist. This brute force on the part of the authorities sparked riots among people who did not want to be treated like criminals.

In 1832, poor people in Liverpool, England—many of them Irish immigrants—became convinced that cholera was a plot by the government to murder the poor. Mobs of people crowded into the streets. They attacked doctors, and threw stones at hospitals. They refused to let doctors examine their sick loved ones.

The fear actually worked in both directions. The poor believed the rich were poisoning them. But the rich also feared the poor. They believed their filthy living environments would eventually contaminate the rich.

Changed Cities

A cholera epidemic had serious economic effects. Sick people went to work less. Dead people did not go to work at all.

Stumbling on the Cure

Ironically, the treatment for cholera was simple, cheap, and available to everyone. In 1831, a young English doctor named William O'Shaughnessy suggested that blood could be "restored" by injecting water and a little salt.

The next year, another doctor, Thomas Latta, tried O'Shaughnessy's solution on an elderly woman. Soon the woman's pulse became stronger. Her breathing got easier. In half an hour, the woman said she felt fine. Unfortunately, after Latta left, the woman's vomiting and diarrhea returned. She did not get more fluids and died. However, Latta wrote that if the therapy had continued, he had "no doubt" she would have survived. He repeated the treatment on more patients. Many of them lived.

Unfortunately, the cure never caught on. The cholera outbreak ended the next year, 1833, making the need for treatment less important. Latta himself died the same year. He did not have much chance to spread his knowledge. Cholera was about to be conquered, but it went into hiding just in time. When it resurfaced in 1847, the cure was lost.

Fearful people stayed out of the streets, depriving merchants of their business. Bakers and butchers, shoemakers and saddle makers—everyone saw their stream of customers dry up. Small business owners scrambled to find money to pay the rent. In England, grocers were hit hard when it was reported that fruits and vegetables offered another way for cholera bacteria to spread.

Officials, wanting to stop the disease's spread, closed public areas like theaters and parks. Hotels were empty. Banks, restaurants, and government offices shut down. Sometimes the closings were not even about fear of spreading the disease. They were ways of stopping immoral activities. By

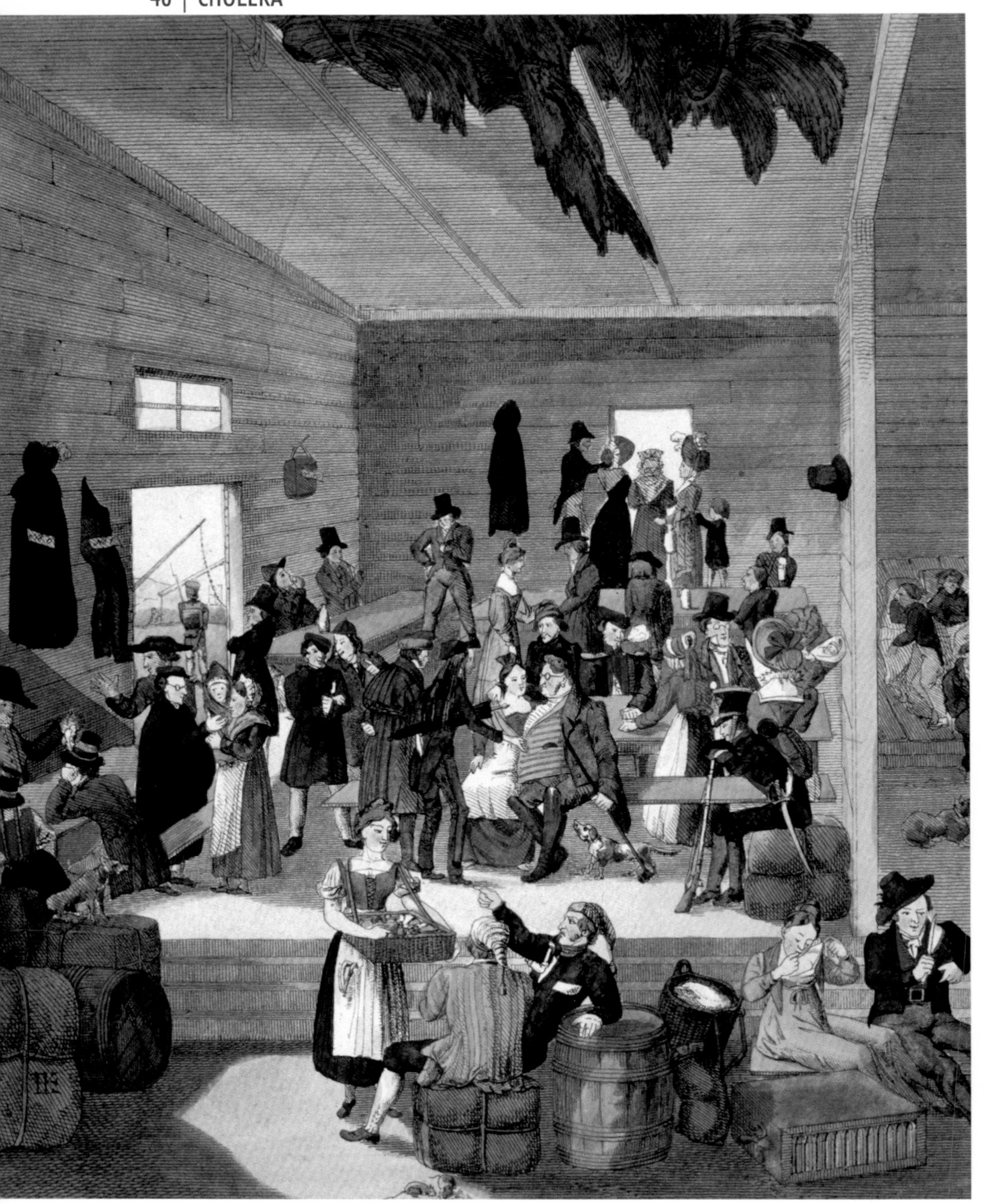

People formed small communities as they waited to be released from quarantine facilities. This 1815 engraving is entitled *Pains and Pleasures of a Cholera Quarantine Station*.

closing bars, people drank alcohol less. Canceling sporting events put the brakes on gambling.

A few services, of course, were in higher demand. The drugstores stayed open. The hospitals stayed open, even though nobody wanted to be admitted. Even with their questionable tactics, doctors stayed busy. And gravediggers stayed very busy.

Quarantines could be an effective weapon against cholera. They might not stop the disease entirely, but they could slow it down. However, quarantines had serious side effects. Rural citizens were largely self-sufficient. They could grow their own food and make a lot of what they needed. City residents, on the other hand, needed contact with the rest of the world. Their economy depended on movement. A quarantine froze all of this activity.

In many cities, residents who could afford to leave did. They fled to smaller towns or the countryside. The streets of New York became deserted in 1832. Broadway, a normally busy street, grew silent. The smallest activity drew attention. If a horse was heard outside, people came to the windows to see what was going on. During that summer, the thriving metropolis of New York—a city of 250,000 people—had grass growing through the cracks in the streets.

In good times, cities brought jobs. But in times of disease, they spread death. Hundreds of thousands of people lived within their boundaries. There was no room for an epidemic.

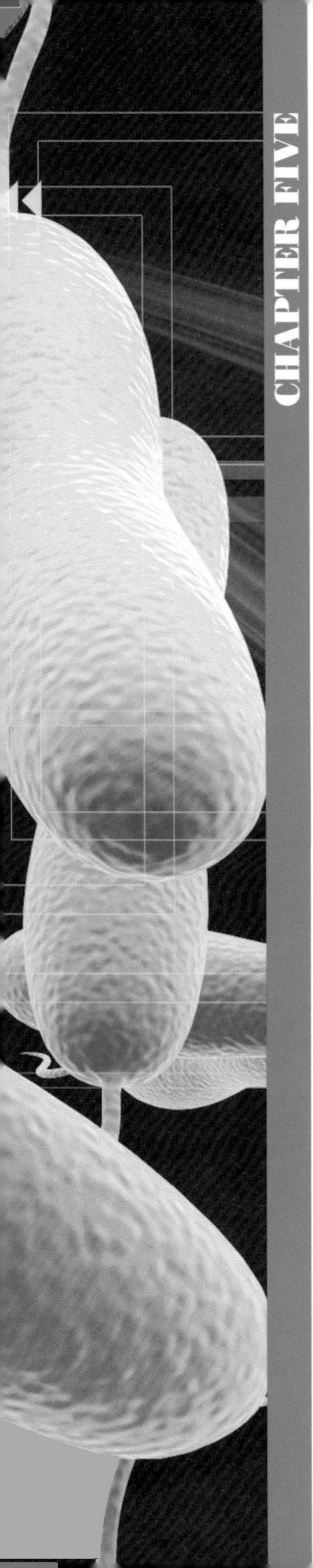

NOBLE EFFORTS

As the disease raged, so did the debate over what to do about it. At the center of the discussion were questions of what caused cholera and how it spread. Nobody had all the answers, but many had part of them. The fight against cholera was a slow process of trying to fit the puzzle pieces together. Through trial and error, insight and luck, people began to strike back.

Looking for a Cause

What was causing the disease? That was the question on everybody's mind, from government officials to scientists to ordinary people living in fear for their lives. The theory of microbes causing disease was not unheard of in the nineteenth century. However, it was not proved. So it was not seriously considered.

Instead, most people, including scientists, believed in the idea of miasmas. Miasmas were clouds of polluted air caused by material that rotted in the soil and water. People thought just the smell alone could cause disease!

Doctors also thought that the same miasma could affect people differently. One person might

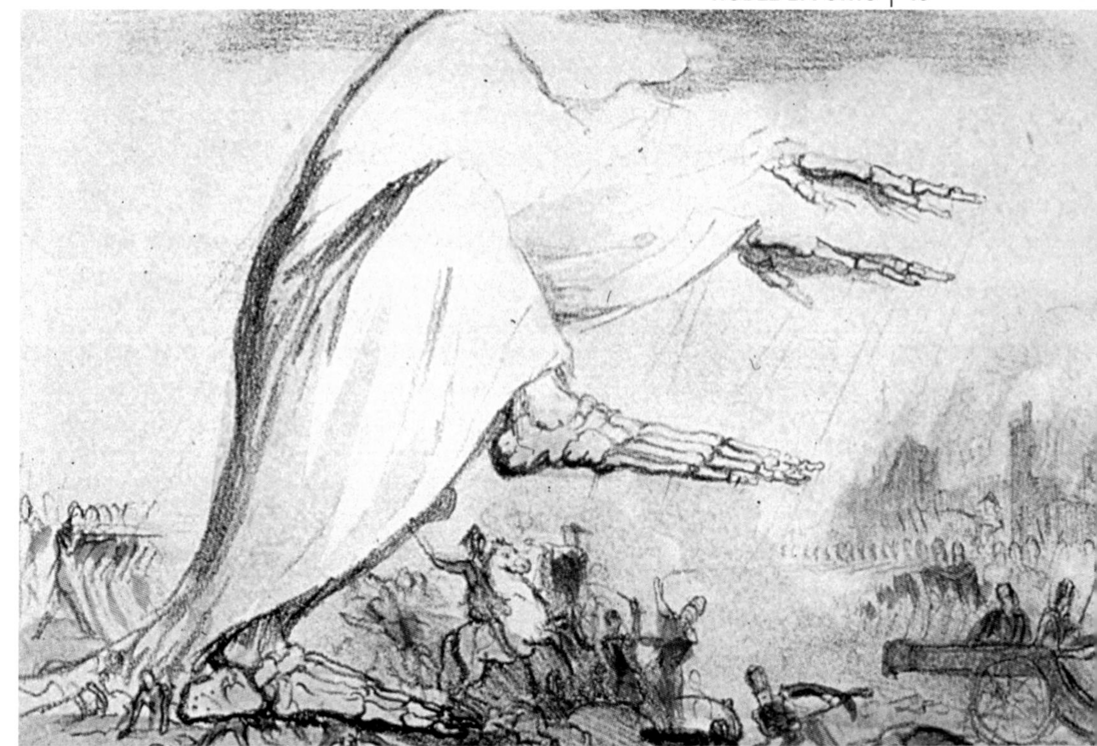

This 1831 drawing pictures cholera as a giant monster that overshadowed even the horrors of war. The disease showed no mercy to people on either side of the conflict.

only suffer from mild diarrhea, while another came down with a full-blown case of cholera. It all depended on the person's natural constitution, as well as his or her physical and mental state at the time.

Only a minority of scientists supported the idea that disease was not generated by miasmas, but could be from another source.

Related to the question of how people got cholera was another mystery: Why?

Anyone who witnessed a cholera epidemic could see that poor people were especially likely to get the disease. Most people concluded that the disease was a result of this poverty. Affluent citizens did not often understand the lives of the poor. They did not trust them. They thought the poor had low moral standards. The misery of cholera was a direct consequence of their behavior. Doctors and public officials stated that laziness and filth were the true sources of disease. These things made poor people weaker. They were less able to fight off disease.

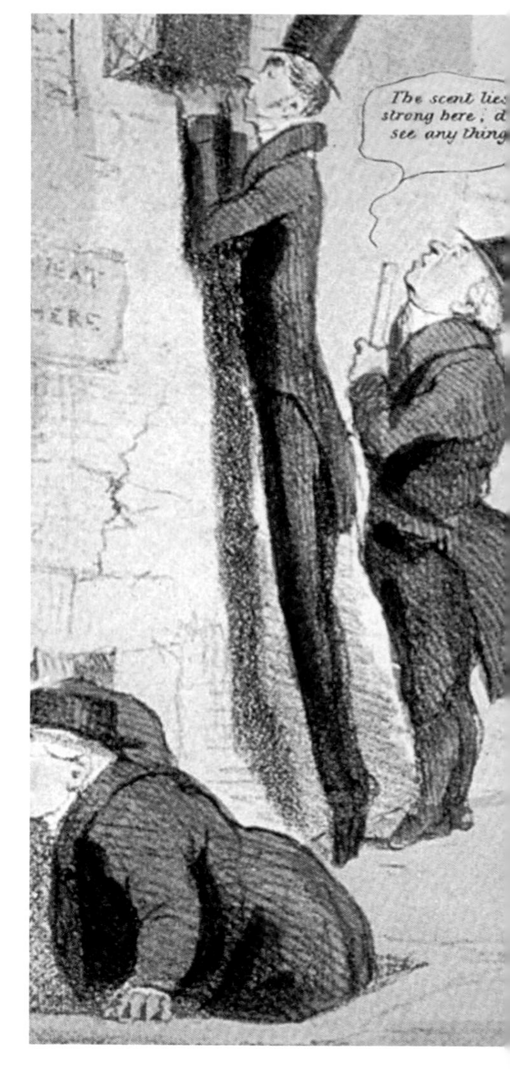

In 1831, the Central Board of Health was formed in England to deal with the epidemic. The board offered the following advice: "The true preventatives [of cholera] are a healthy body and a cheerful unruffled mind."

Many people believed God sent cholera as punishment. An epidemic would cleanse the population of people who did not have good morals. Historian Charles Rosenberg wrote that people believed "cholera was a scourge not of mankind, but of the sinner."

In fact, poor people were not any more sinful or lazy than anyone else. They were just poor. They often did not have proper clothing or a warm place to sleep. They might not even have enough to eat.

The accusation that the poor lived in filth was often true. They had no way to get rid of it, and they could not afford to live anywhere else. The physical strain on their bodies, combined with living in conditions that bred disease, made the

Positively we must find something; it wont do to lose our Twenty guineas a day
CHOLERA MORBUS
Oh! if I can but find a smell
ooseness of the bowels the beginning of the Cholera

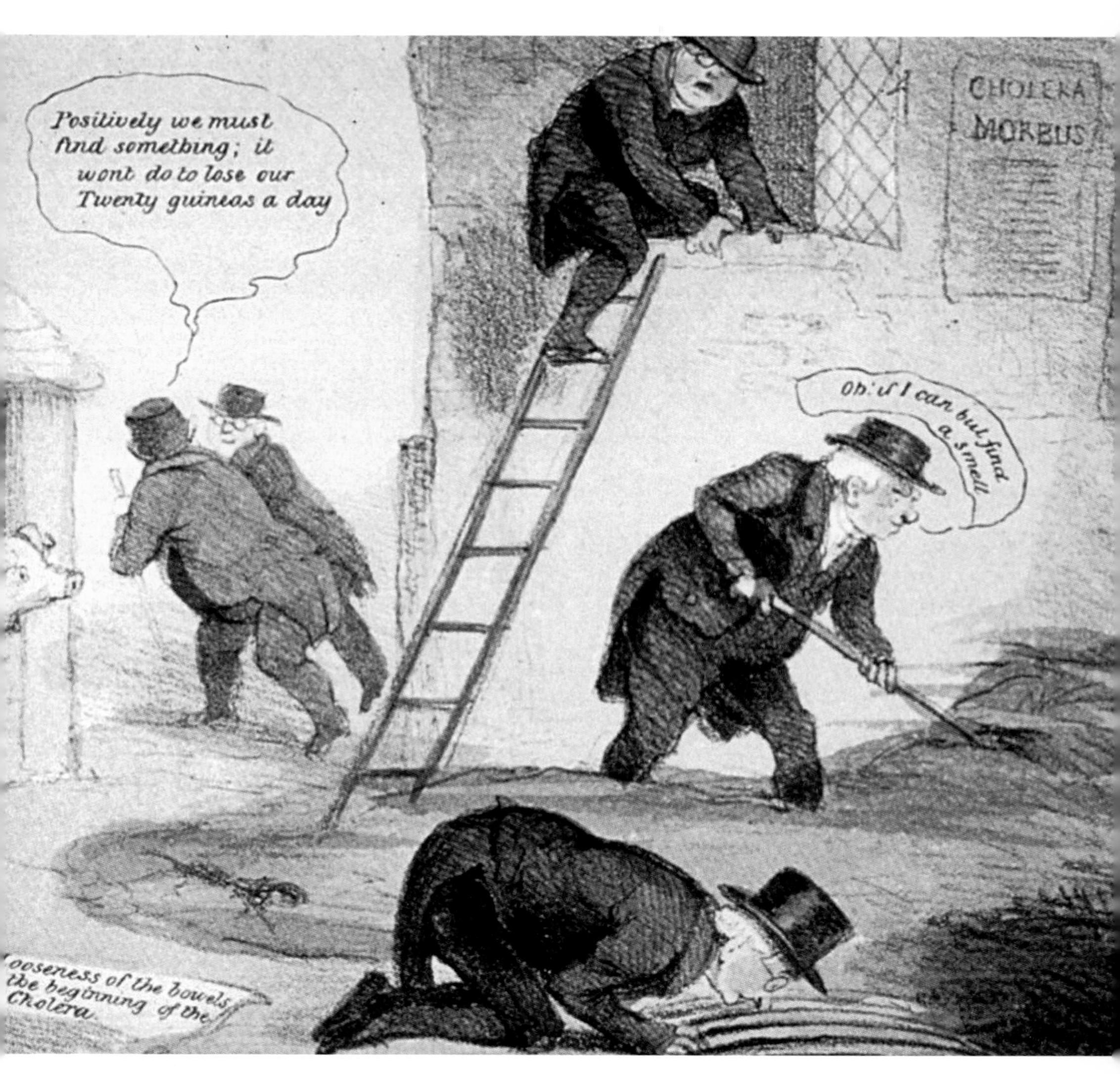

Members of England's Board of Health search for cases of cholera in this caricature from 1832. The board was not successful in stopping the disease.

rate of cholera much higher among the poor. But it wasn't a lack of morality that put them at risk. It was a lack of money.

In the Water

Although most scientists believed in miasmas, one London doctor believed something else. John Snow had observed cholera patients and formed a different theory. He didn't believe cholera spread through the air. Instead, he thought it moved through water.

In 1849, cholera came to London, giving Snow a chance to test his theory. He found out that in one neighborhood where people were sick, residents got their water from a well that sometimes overflowed. The water would wash down the street, pick up whatever was laying around, and then flow back down into the well. To Snow, this was proof that contaminated water was causing cholera. Still, he wanted more evidence.

Another neighborhood experienced an outbreak. The official explanation was a miasma caused by overflowing cesspools. But Snow took a sample of the drinking water and found a grape peel. He realized it was a bit of undigested food. In other words, it had already passed through a person. Wastewater had mixed with the drinking water. Finally, Snow was convinced. He furiously went to work writing and publishing his results.

His discoveries were largely ignored, but Snow kept collecting evidence. Several companies provided London's water. In 1853, one company switched to using water from a much cleaner part of the Thames River. Snow gathered data that showed people who drank this water were much less likely to get cholera.

When the Broad Street outbreak occurred in London in 1854, Snow was able to test his theory once again. He researched the cases, painstakingly making a map showing

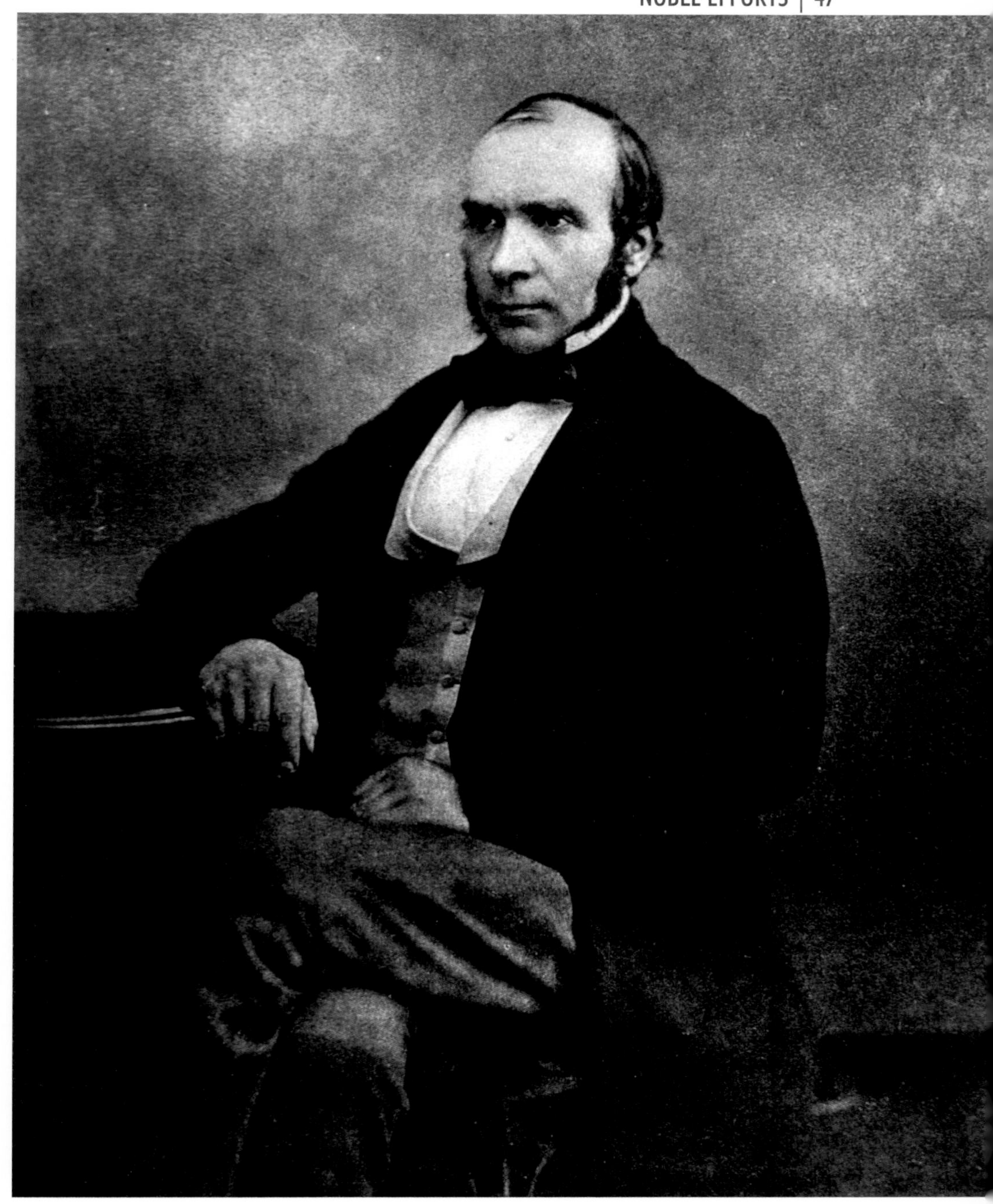

John Snow helped discover the cause of cholera but died at age forty-five, before his efforts had made a difference. He devoted his life to medicine, also doing much research in the field of anesthesia.

where the sick people lived. Case by case, he traced them back to the Broad Street pump. Snow's experiments kept showing him the same thing. Cholera was always linked to water.

In 1866, East London experienced a large outbreak. Snow had died by this time. A London official named William Farr investigated. Farr had previously worked with Snow, but he did not believe in his theories. This time, however, Farr saw the proof. He traced one person after another to the same polluted water.

A City Steps Up

By the time cholera came to New York in the 1860s, people had accepted that there was a link between sanitation and

Edwin Chadwick and the Sewers

Edwin Chadwick was a doer. He saw how London's poor lived in squalid environments. He was convinced this was the reason they got sick so much. His mission was to clean up London. Chadwick was not a particularly likable man, but he was determined and committed. His beliefs, from a scientific point of view, were not entirely wrong. Human waste did cause disease. However, Chadwick did not believe the waste was dangerous because of any microscopic life it might contain. Instead, he believed the odor poisoned the air and made people sick. As he put it, "All smell is disease." He felt the answer was to install a sewer system. It would carry the waste out of the city and dump it into the Thames River.

Chadwick's intentions were good. But we now know his solution was terribly harmful. By emptying waste into the river, the sewers contaminated Londoners' main source of drinking water. In the years following Chadwick's new sewer systems, the city's cholera outbreaks only got worse.

sickness. Although they did not fully understand how it worked, the evidence was overwhelming. People who lived in filthy environments got sick much more often.

In 1865, the citizens of New York put together a report listing the city's sanitary failings—and there were many. The next year, the Metropolitan Board of Health was formed. New Yorkers feared that cholera was on its way again. They wanted to protect themselves as much as possible. In a little over two months, the board's staff poured through New York's filthy streets. They issued more than 7,500 citations for things that needed to be cleaned up. The police got in on the action, too. They formed a special group of officers who helped enforce the board's orders.

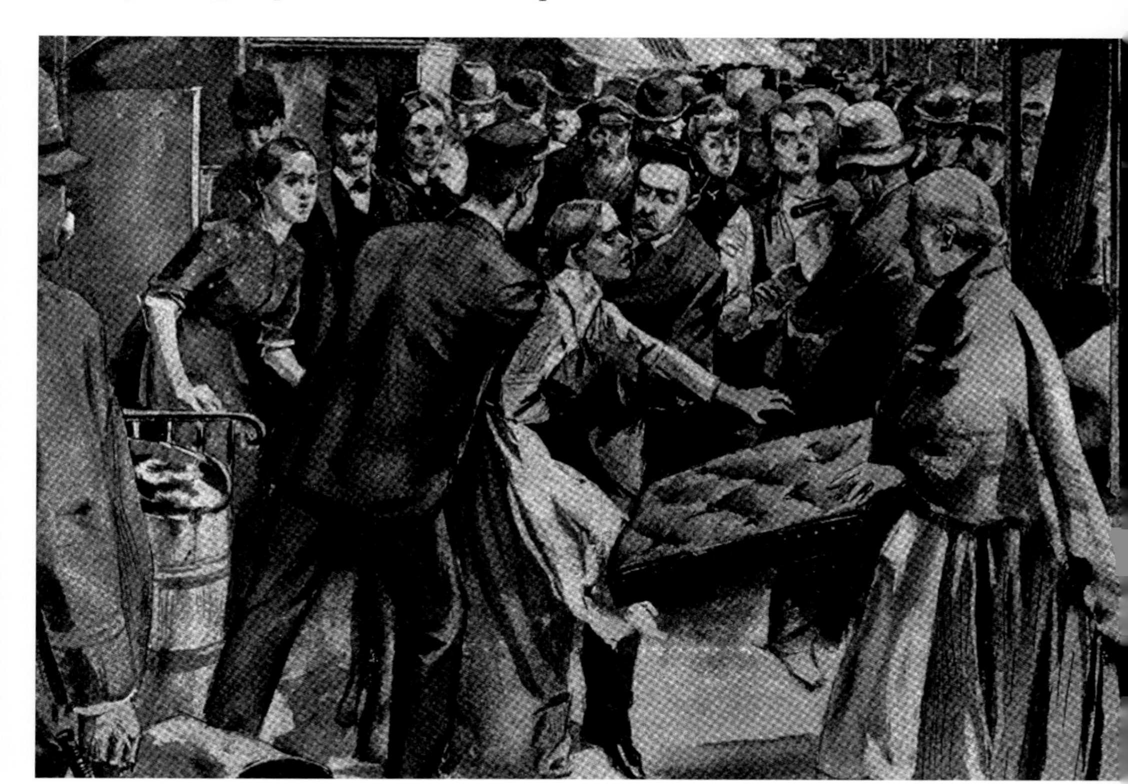

A crowd watches as a woman is helped into an ambulance in this 1892 drawing. Cholera victims were often afraid to go to hospitals because so many people died there.

Despite the cleaning craze, cholera arrived in New York by April 1866. It was not unexpected, however, and New Yorkers were more prepared than they had ever been. This time, they did everything they could to stop its spread.

When a case was reported, the information was telegraphed to a central office. The wheels of bureaucracy began to turn. The personal belongings of cholera patients, such as clothes, sheets, and pillows, were burned. The home and the surrounding areas were disinfected. Any other inhabitants were quickly moved to hospital tents. The board even had small amounts of an "anti-cholera mixture" prepared and distributed to police stations throughout the city. Whether the mixture actually worked or not is questionable, but it took effort and organization even to try. New Yorkers were serious about fighting cholera, and this time, they won the battle.

When the epidemic ended, the number of people who died was only 10 percent of what it had been in 1849. The Metropolitan Board of Health had done its job.

TEN GREAT QUESTIONS *to ask* SOMEONE WHO WORKS FOR THE BOARD OF HEALTH

1. What can I do to avoid contracting cholera while traveling to other countries?
2. How many cases of cholera are reported per year?
3. What are my chances of catching cholera?
4. Is there a cholera vaccine?
5. What are the long-term effects of having cholera?
6. How is cholera diagnosed?
7. What are the chances of a cholera outbreak where I live?
8. What can I do to help prevent the spread of cholera?
9. How does someone pursue a career in disease prevention?
10. What is being done to prevent outbreaks of other diseases?

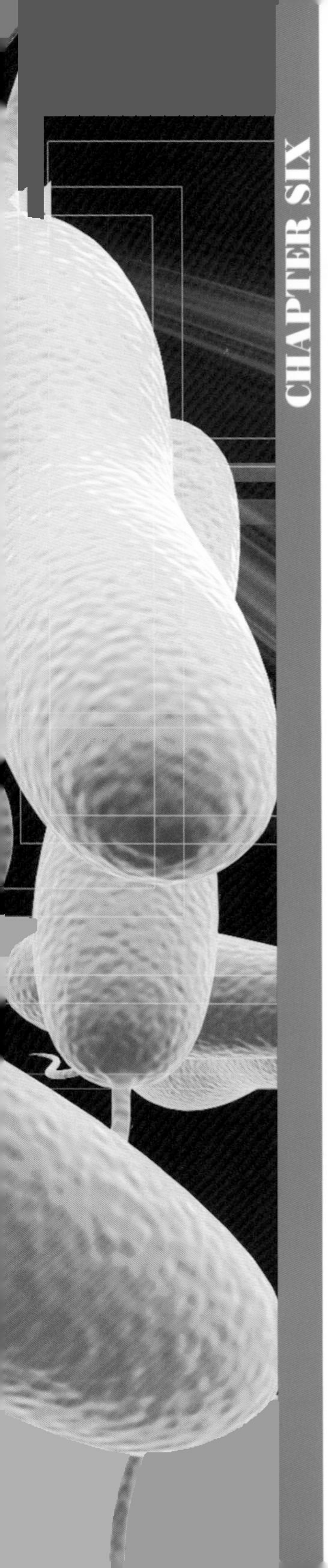

CHAPTER SIX

STEPS FORWARD STEPS BACK

By the late nineteenth century, the world's cities were beginning to solve the problems of growing populations. Staying healthy meant staying clean. Cholera had not vanished, however. It was especially a problem in developing areas in Latin America, Asia, and Africa.

A Killer Comma

In 1854, John Snow conducted his famous Broad Street investigation. That same year, an Italian scientist named Filippo Pacini actually viewed the cholera bacterium under a microscope. Pacini was a firm believer in germ theory, but the majority of scientists, who still believed in miasmas, scoffed at his views. Probably because of this, Pacini's research remained unknown. Snow doubtless would have welcomed information that confirmed his theories, but he never knew about Pacini's discovery.

Neither did Robert Koch. Koch is the scientist who got credit for discovering the cholera bacterium almost thirty years later. In 1883, he was in Egypt during a cholera outbreak, working with a team of French scientists. He noticed the bacterium in the diarrhea of cholera patients.

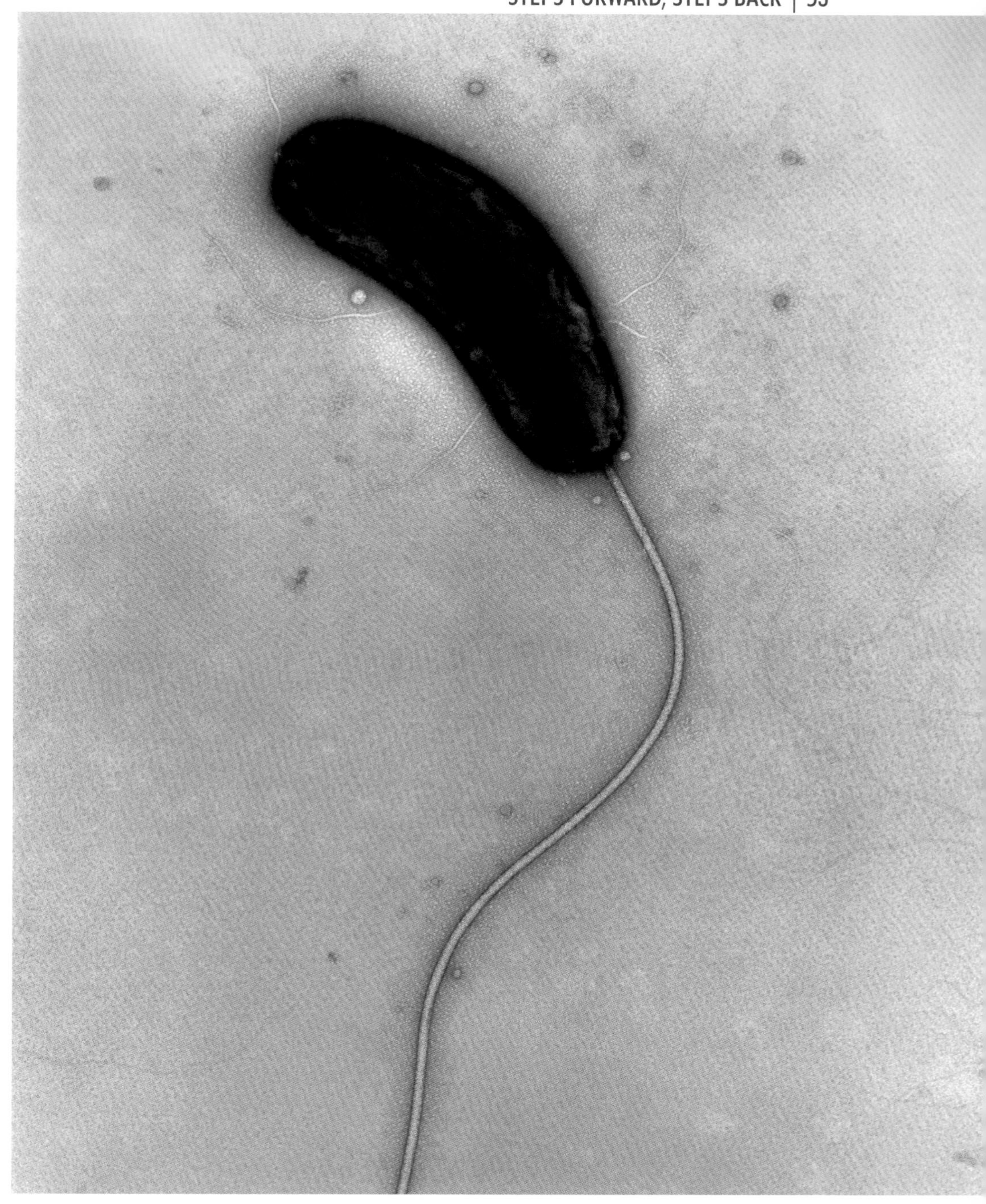

In this magnified image, the tail of the cholera bacterium, called a flagellum, can be seen. The bacterium gets its name, *Vibrio cholerae*, because it appears to vibrate.

He also noticed that it was not present in the stools of people who were not sick with cholera. Koch believed he had found what caused the disease.

The bacterium is shaped like a thick rod, resembling a pickle. Koch described it as being "a little bent, like a comma." Koch was a well-respected scientist. During his career, he also discovered the bacteria that cause tuberculosis and anthrax. For his work, he was awarded the Nobel Prize for Physiology or Medicine. Pacini's work on cholera had gone unnoticed, but the medical world paid attention to Robert Koch. Because of his discovery, the theories of miasma finally began to fade. (Pacini's work was formally recognized in 1965.)

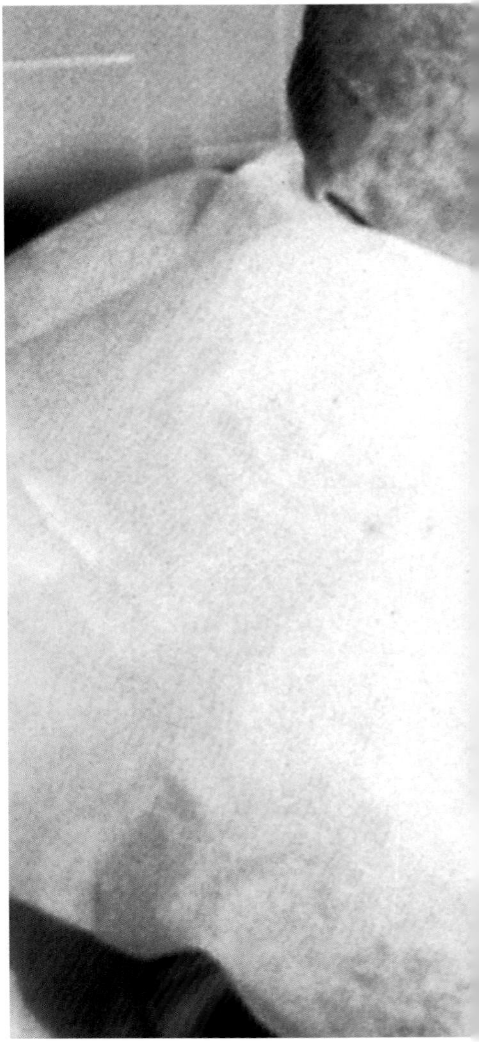

Cholera in Naples

By the late 1800s, the cholera bacterium had been identified. The link between hygiene and health had been made. Cities had launched efforts to protect their citizens from cholera. It was finally recognized as a disease, not a result of moral weakness. But it was not conquered, and the fear of it remained.

In 1884, cholera came to Naples, a city in southern Italy. People reacted in the same ways they had during previous epidemics. They were scared. They did not trust doctors or the authorities. Citizens of Naples felt the government usually

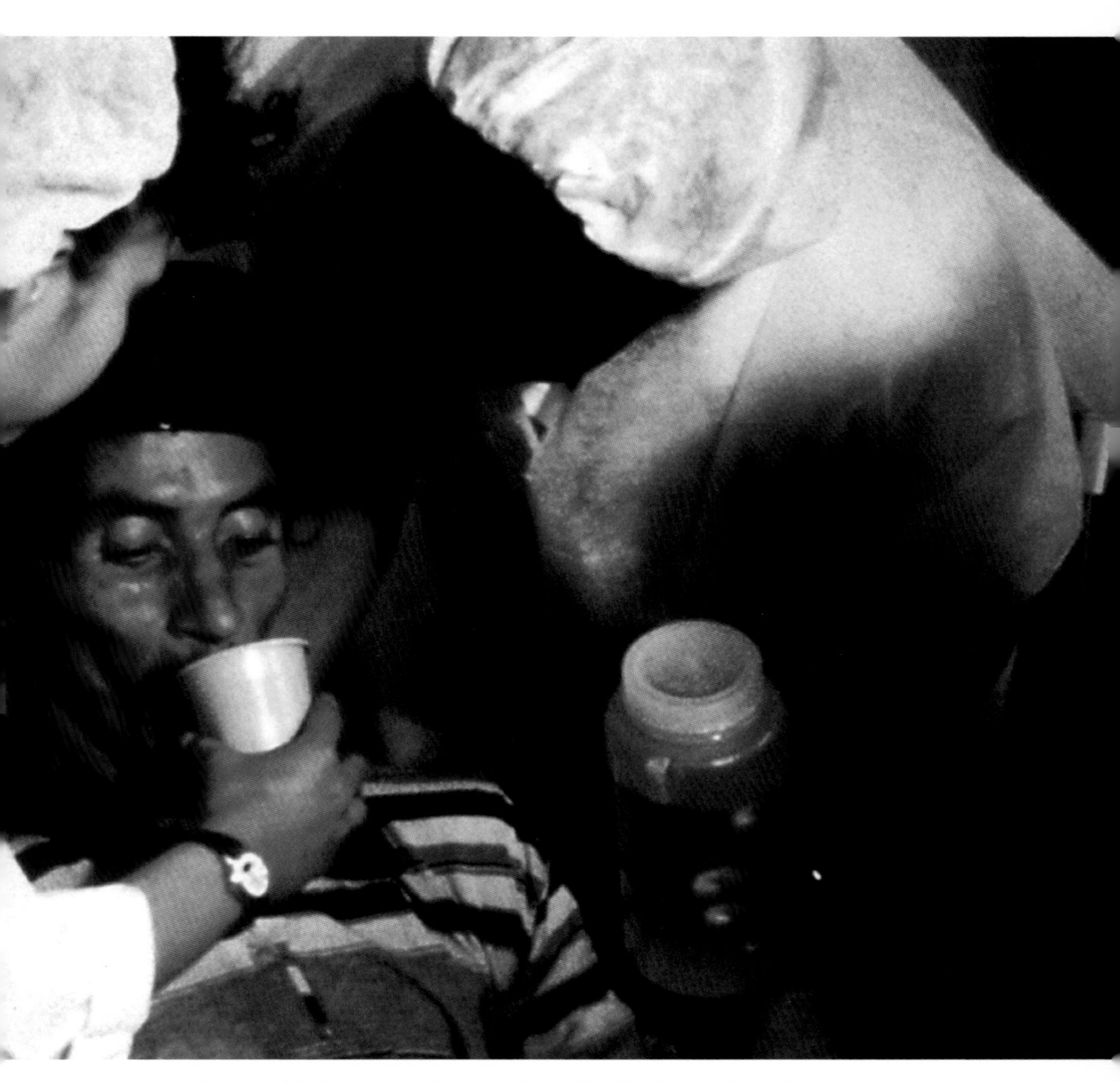

A nurse offers a drink to a cholera patient. Oral rehydration therapy (a solution of water, salt, and sugar) is extremely effective in treating cholera, but it did not become widely used until the mid-1900s.

ignored them. Then when cholera broke out, officials swooped in. They cleaned up and handed out medicine, but the cholera only got worse. People became more distrustful than ever.

Naples was one of Italy's most important port cities. Italian officials decided it was important to make Naples a safe place. After the epidemic, the Italian government decided to tear down much of the city and then rebuild it to make it more resistant to disease. New buildings would be shorter and spaced farther apart, letting in more air and sunlight to streets and residences. Streets were positioned so that wind would blow through them, pushing out any bad miasmas that might try to build up. (Despite Koch's discovery, the idea of miasmas was still strong in 1884.)

Buildings would be constructed on higher ground to protect them from decaying soil that produced miasmas. A sewer system would drain the soil, and new pipes would feed water into it. (Ironically, the new water supply was only designed to flush the sewers; it did not bring fresh water to individual residences.) To top it all off, there would be a new hospital.

As with most ambitious projects, this one experienced problems from the start. Costs added up. Arguments ate up time and money. Contractors did not follow through with their jobs. The new and improved city of Naples emerged only half finished. Also, what had been done came at a high price—and it wasn't only money. The rebuilding had also forced people out of their homes.

For all the trouble they had been through, residents were expecting a new, disease-proof city. If cholera returned, officials knew they would be under the microscope. Would the population of Naples be able to withstand the disease?

In 1910, cholera did return. The answer was obvious: Naples was not able to resist an outbreak. Officials, however, refused to admit the problem. The government lied about

Drinking Death

Even after Robert Koch identified the cholera bacterium, the idea of miasmas took time to die. Max Pettenkofer was a German scientist who worked hard to improve sanitation and help prevent cholera. But he believed in miasmas, not bacteria.

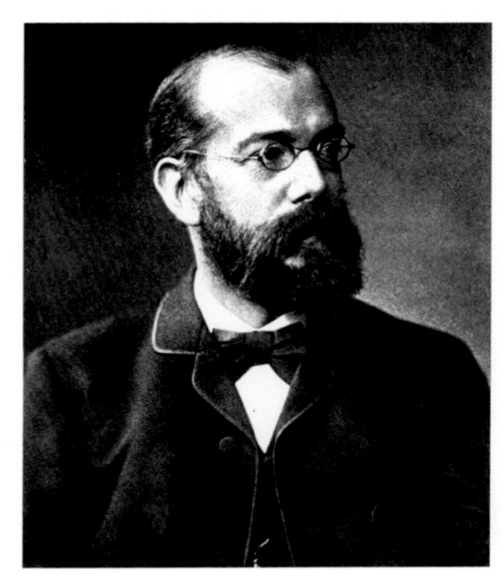

German doctor Robert Koch was one of the first people to study bacteria and their role in disease.

He asked Koch to send him a sample of the cholera bacteria. In a dramatic gesture, Pettenkofer drank the contents of the flask in front of a room full of people. He did not develop cholera, and he certainly did not die. He believed he had proved his point. He wrote a letter to Koch, reporting that he was "happy to be able to inform [Koch] that he remains in his usual good health." What spared Pettenkofer? Not everyone who ingests cholera bacteria gets sick. Also, he had suffered from an attack of cholera several years before. It's possible that he had developed some resistance.

sanitary conditions. It ordered the press not to report any problems. It even refused to inform doctors about what was going on. Naples' officials had to choose between two undesirable choices. They could admit the presence of cholera and risk the economic well-being of the city. Or they could deny it and risk public health because they could not inform people of what was going on. They chose the second option. Officially, cholera did not exist in Naples. In reality, thousands of people were dying.

Information leaked out, of course. But for the most part, the government succeeded in its cover-up. The Italian newspapers did not break their silence until the epidemic was almost over.

"Cholera Cures Itself"

In 1960, a U.S. Army doctor stated, "Cholera cures itself, like a common cold." The catch, he added, was in keeping the

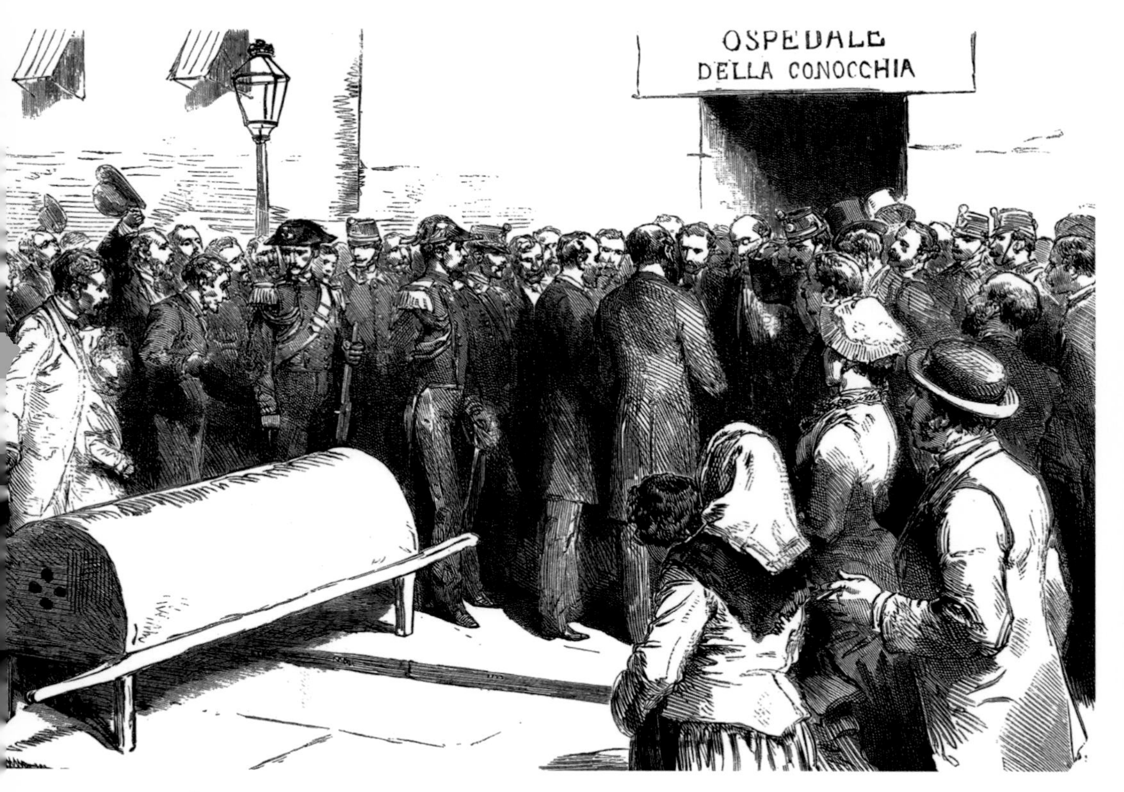

Government officials visit a hospital during the 1884 cholera outbreak in Naples, Italy. Authorities were not able to stop the disease from spreading.

patient alive while this was happening. There really is no cure for cholera except time. But there is a treatment, and that is what Robert Allan Phillips studied. Rehydration (water replacement) therapy had been tried as far back as the 1830s, but then it vanished.

Finally, in 1960, Phillips brought the treatment into the public eye. During World War II, he had developed a way to replace bodily fluids in wounded soldiers. Then in 1947, while working at a medical research facility in Cairo, Egypt, he found himself in the middle of a cholera epidemic. Building on his previous research, Phillips developed an oral rehydration therapy. Basically, this came down to drinking a solution of water that was mixed with a little bit of salt and sugar. (The salt and sugar help the body absorb the water.)

Today, antibiotics such as tetracycline can also be given to cholera patients. These medicines on their own (without rehydration) do not cure cholera. However, they can make the length of the illness shorter. A downside to antibiotics is that over time the bacteria become used to the drugs and more resistant to them. This is already happening.

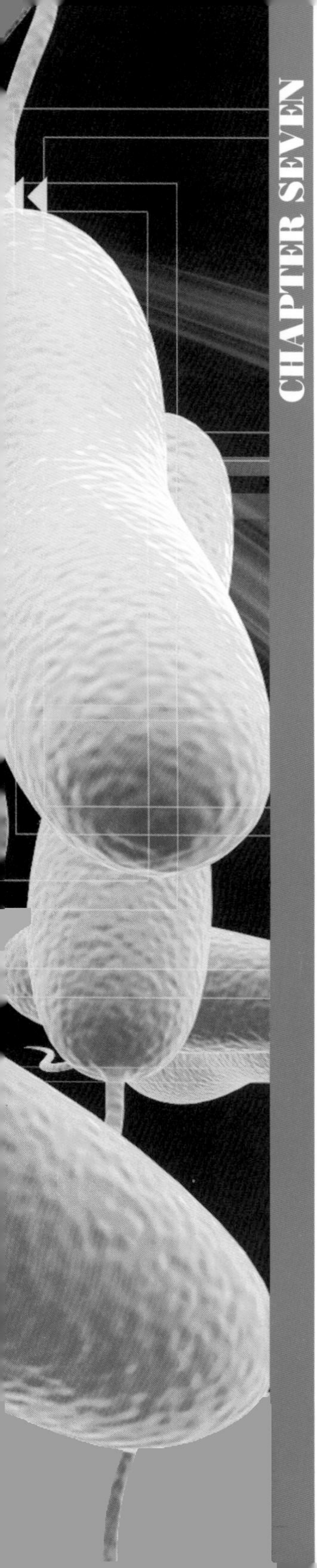

LOOKING FORWARD

Clean water: It's the one ingredient needed for both the prevention and treatment of cholera. However, getting clean water remains a problem in many parts of the world. Cholera still sickens and kills thousands of people worldwide. The challenge for today is much the same as it was 150 years ago. People need the tools to fight the disease, since it's not going away.

A Changing Disease

After going into hibernation for nearly forty years, cholera returned in 1961. This time, it had gotten a makeover. Instead of the traditional cholera bacterium, this one was a new strain. It was called El Tor, after the place in Indonesia where it began. The El Tor strain infects more people—without making them sick—than the classic strain. It's also a better survivor. These factors made it easier for it to spread unnoticed. Outbreaks occurred throughout the 1960s and 1970s in Africa, Asia, and Russia. In 1991, an outbreak started in Peru and then spread throughout Latin America. More than a million people came down with cholera, and about ten thousand died. In 1992, still another strain was identified.

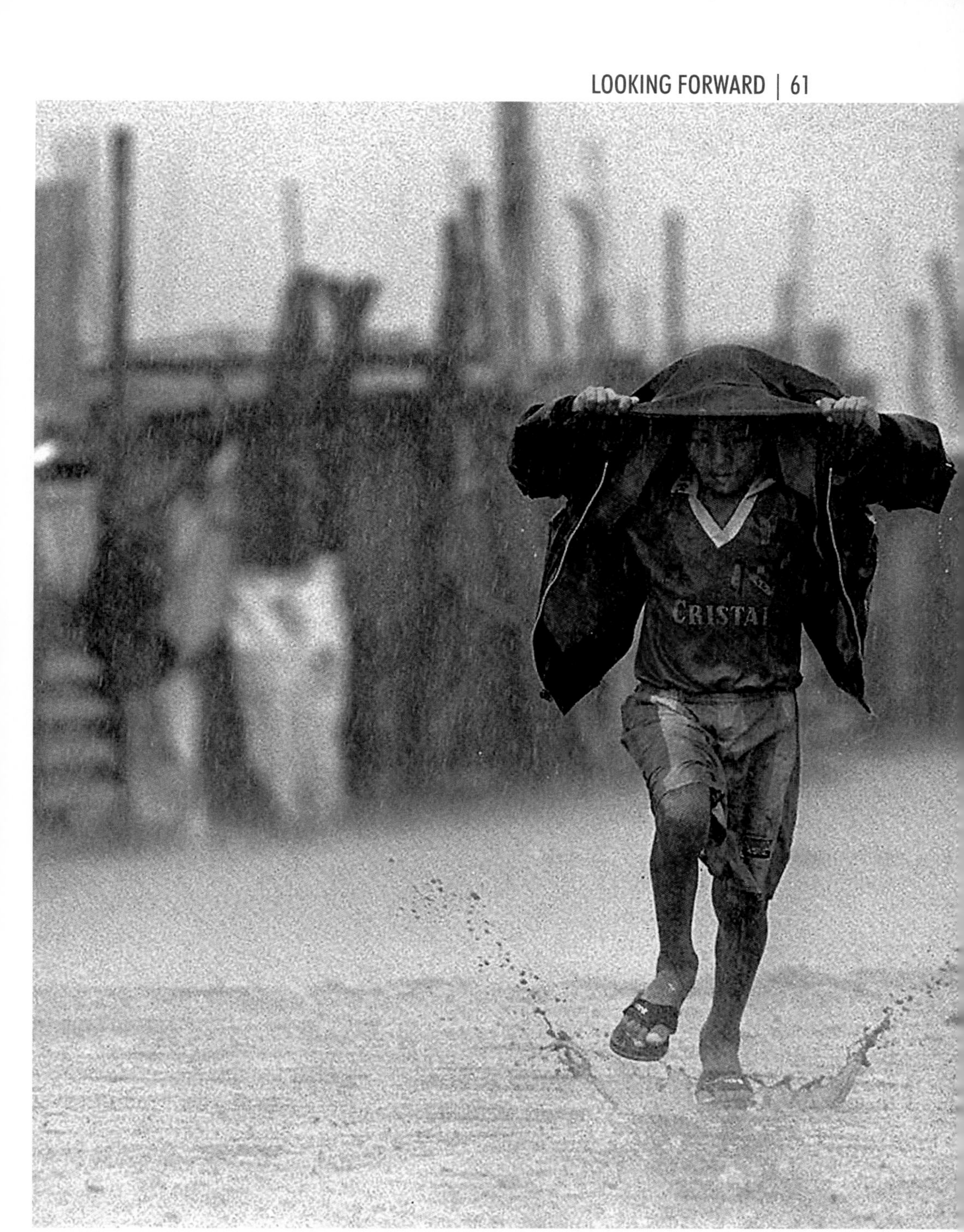

A boy runs through the rain in Tuman, Peru, in South America. Flooding can overwhelm drainage systems and cause unsanitary conditions that may lead to cholera outbreaks.

The 1990s epidemic in South America showed that many people still were at risk for cholera. It also dredged up old attitudes. In the nineteenth century, poor people and immigrants had been blamed for the spread of cholera. A researcher in Venezuela observed a similar trend this time around. Poor people and native populations were blamed for this outbreak of cholera. It was not only because of their lack of sanitation. They were also blamed because their cultures were different.

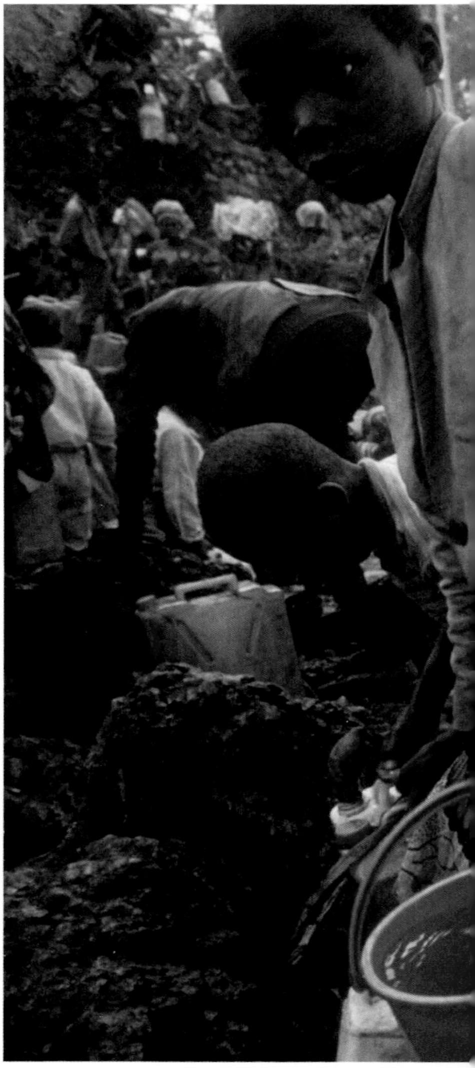

Recent Outbreaks

In the early 1990s, the African country of Rwanda was in upheaval. Civil war was tearing it apart. Hundreds of thousands of citizens fled the country. Many of them ended up in nearby Goma, Zaire, huddled together at a large, outdoor camp. These refugees needed food, clothing, shelter, medical care, and protection. And they badly needed water.

The town of Goma sits on top of volcanic rock—hardened lava. The ground is too hard to drill wells. There were far too many refugees to import enough water on trucks. The only source of water was a large lake called Lake Kivu, located near the emergency camp.

There was nowhere to dispose of waste properly. And with more than one hundred thousand people, there was a lot of waste.

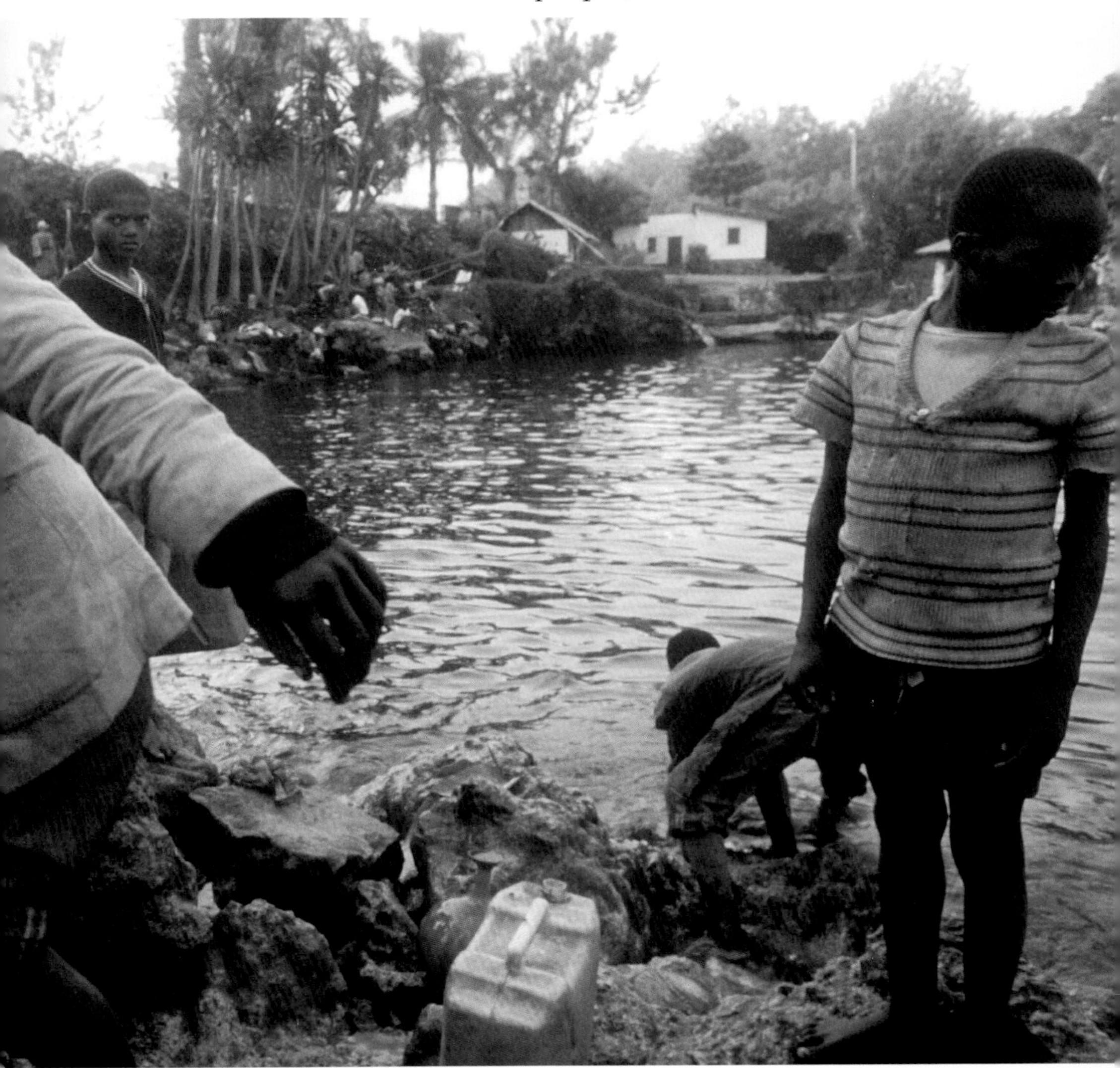

In 1994, war refugees from Rwanda camped near Lake Kivu, which was their only source of water. The lake became polluted with human waste and caused a cholera outbreak that killed thousands.

Much of it drained into Lake Kivu, where people were getting their drinking water. Within days, cholera broke out. Disease and death spread ruthlessly among refugees who were trapped with no clean water and nowhere to go. The sick were lucky if they could even get to one of the tents set up to provide medical care. Corpses were stacked by the side of the road.

During a single day in July 1994, six thousand people died. In a month, that number had climbed to sixty thousand. It was the worst outbreak of a waterborne disease in history. Recent years have seen more outbreaks. In 2007, about 4,500 people in Iraq became sick from cholera. About two dozen of them died. In 2008, Iraq reported more cases, as did Vietnam.

Simple Solutions

Cholera has a low-tech treatment: drink fluids. Now it's getting some low-tech prevention as well. Many areas don't have sophisticated water treatment facilities, but that might be OK. Cholera bacteria can live inside tiny animals called zooplankton, which live in water. Rita Colwell, a U.S. scientist who studies cholera, knew that removing the zooplankton from the water would make it safer. Saris are long cloths worn by women throughout India and South Asia. Colwell experimented with folding a sari cloth several times and filtering water through it. This simple process worked. The number of infections decreased in people who drank this water.

Another solution came from American inventor Dean Kamen. He made a machine that will take any kind of water and purify it through evaporation. It will even clean up raw sewage! The machines are about the size of a dishwasher. They do not need filters or chemicals to work. As a bonus, they generate electricity at the same time. One machine can produce about 1,000 liters (1,056 quarts) of water per day. The best part is the machine's fuel—it runs on animal or human waste.

In August 2008, a major outbreak came to Zimbabwe, Africa. The epidemic continued into 2009. About a hundred thousand people were infected, and there were more than four thousand deaths.

Zimbabwe's government was having problems. Officials battled over politics and the economy. Meanwhile, civil services like garbage collection were ignored. The economic crisis made health care unreliable. Doctors and nurses refused to work because they were not getting paid. Patients were being asked to pay huge fees for their treatment. There was not enough medicine to go around. There were no mysteries about the disease this time around, but it still spread. It was not a medical problem, but a social one.

Effects of Climate

Wars, poverty, and a lack of social services all contribute to cholera outbreaks. But what about nature?

Most scientists believe that global warming is getting worse. Cholera bacteria like warm water. Hotter temperatures mean the polar ice caps could melt faster, raising sea levels all over the world. This could lead to severe flooding, especially along the coasts. Drainage systems could be overwhelmed. Fresh water could get contaminated by sewage. And cholera could easily take hold.

Warmer temperatures may also affect ocean currents. Water that is full of nutrients usually sits at the bottom of the ocean. Now it could rise to the top. Plankton—tiny plants and animals—now have plenty to eat. As their populations increase, so does the cholera bacteria.

Even air temperatures play a part. A study conducted from 2003 to 2006 showed that when the thermometer rose, the number of people infected with cholera also rose—by almost 5 percent.

The 1991 outbreak in Peru was tied to El Niño, a weather pattern that causes temperatures to rise in the ocean off the

SHELF COMPANIES
The Herald
Cholera hits city suburbs
Preventive measures against cholera
Teenager accused of raping niece's daughters
AU official calls for speedy resolution of conflicts
WE ALSO DELIVER
NEW
Real Quality
Real Price Beater
Real Bread
VIVON

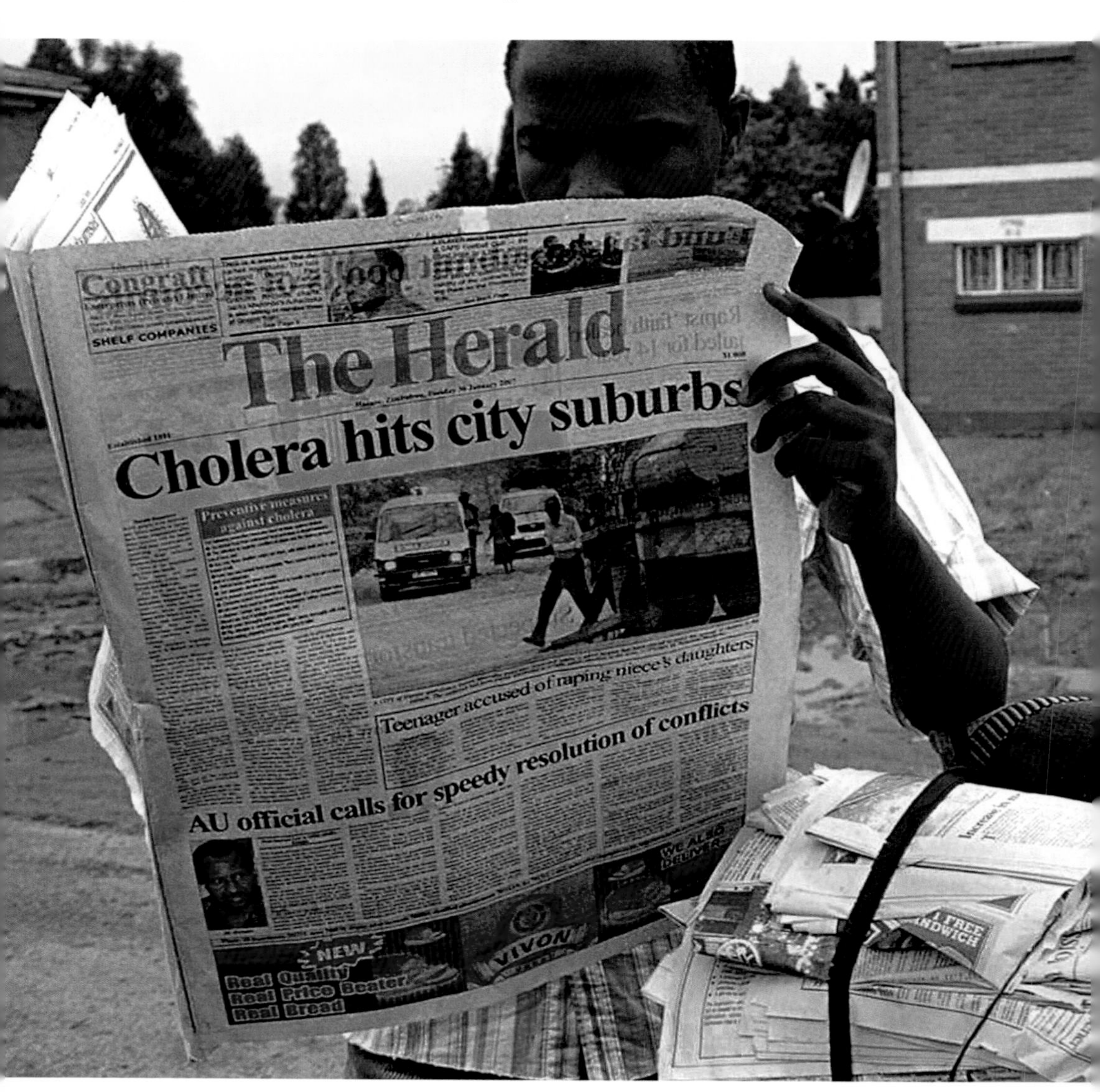

A man reads about a cholera outbreak in the African country of Zimbabwe. In 2009, about a hundred thousand people came down with cholera after civil services collapsed.

west coast of South America. Studies have shown that cholera epidemics get worse after El Niño has been around. Because of global warming, El Niño is likely to get stronger, meaning that cholera itself could become more common.

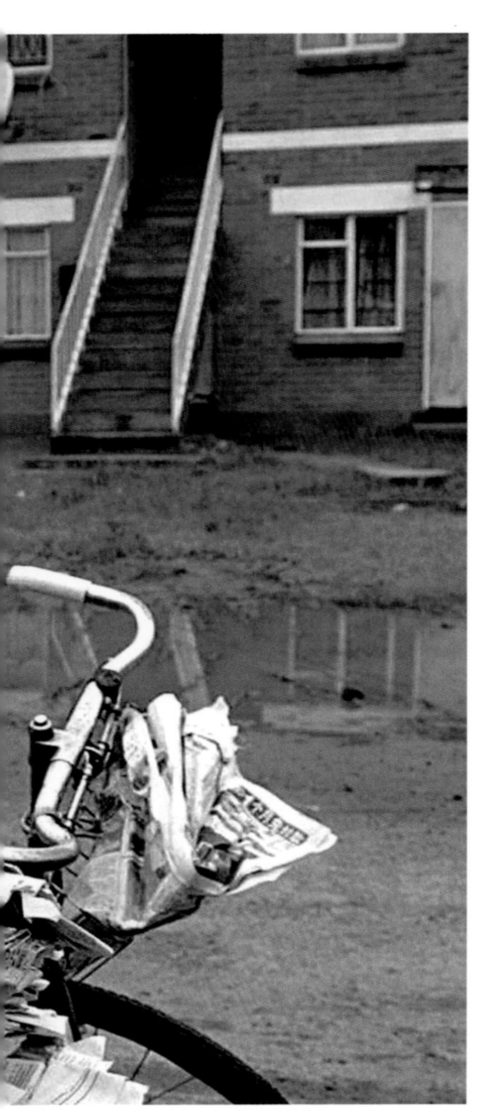

A bright spot is that scientists can use satellite imaging to track rising oceans and warmer water temperatures. These pictures show where an outbreak of cholera might occur. This can give people a warning so that they will be ready to fight cholera.

The Future

Although many countries around the world provide safe water for their citizens, there are many more that don't. Wars and poverty in areas throughout Africa, Asia, and South America mean millions of people don't have clean water or basic sanitary services, such as toilets.

Educating the public about cholera is an important part of fighting the disease. So is making sure doctors have the information and resources they need. Unfortunately, it is human nature to ignore things until they become problems. Sometimes it takes an outbreak to get things moving.

It was during an epidemic in 1854 that John Snow made his famous map that helped prove the source of the disease. Now the tools are even better. With current technology and the power of the Internet, scientists and government agencies can track where problems are occurring around the world.

Communication. Education. Technology. All of these play a part in the battle against cholera. Right now, the struggle goes on. The world is changing, and cholera is changing with it. Doctors, scientists, and governments have not conquered it yet. However, they can fight. And someday, King Cholera may no longer rule.

GLOSSARY

affluent Financially well-off.

antibiotic A substance or compound that kills or inhibits the reproduction of bacteria.

autopsy The study or dissection of a corpse to learn the cause of death and information about bodily processes.

bacteria Unicellular microorganisms; some are capable of causing infectious disease, but most are actually a necessary part of human life.

coincide To happen at the same time.

dehydrated Having lost excessive amounts of water, or not having enough water.

dredge To dig up; expose.

endemic Naturally occurring.

epidemic The occurrence of a disease beyond what is normal.

fasting Not eating for a certain period of time, often for spiritual reasons.

microbe An organism that is microscopic.

outbreak An occurrence of a disease greater than would be expected in a particular time and place.

pandemic The occurrence of a disease that spreads across an entire region or worldwide, larger than an epidemic.

pathogen An infectious agent or germ.

purge To expel; to get rid of.

quarantine The practice of isolating sick people from healthy people.

ravage To cause destruction and pain.

refugee A person who has been displaced from his or her home, usually because of war.

scoff To dismiss in a scornful way.

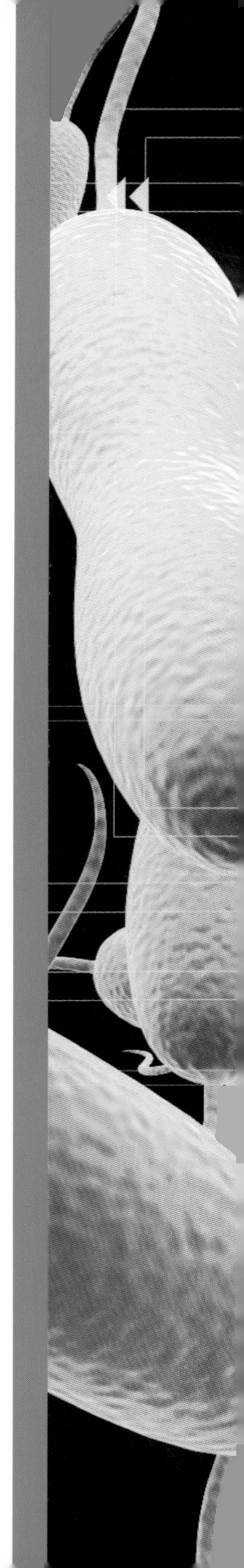

scourge A widespread occurrence of something that causes pain.
shun To refuse to associate with someone; to actively avoid or ignore.
squalid Extremely dirty.
susceptible More likely to be affected by something.
thrive To grow or flourish; to do exceptionally well.
toxin A poisonous substance produced by living cells or organisms.
vital Necessary; extremely important.

FOR MORE INFORMATION

Center for the History of Global Health and Disease
History of Medicine
Johns Hopkins University
School of Medicine
Welch Library, 3rd Floor
1900 East Monument Street
Baltimore, MD 21205-2113
(410) 955-3178
Web site: http://www.hopkinsmedicine.org/histmed/programs/history_disease
Programs at this center focus on studying the history of diseases from both medical and social perspectives.

Centers for Disease Control and Prevention (CDC)
1600 Clifton Road
Atlanta, GA 30333
(800) 232-4636
Web site: http://www.cdc.gov
The CDC collects and maintains information on diseases affecting people worldwide, as well as provides resources to combat disease.

Howard Hughes Medical Institute
4000 Jones Bridge Road
Chevy Chase, MD 20815-6789
(301) 215-8500
Web site: http://www.hhmi.org
This nonprofit organization does biomedical research and supports science education. Its Web site includes a special section for children.

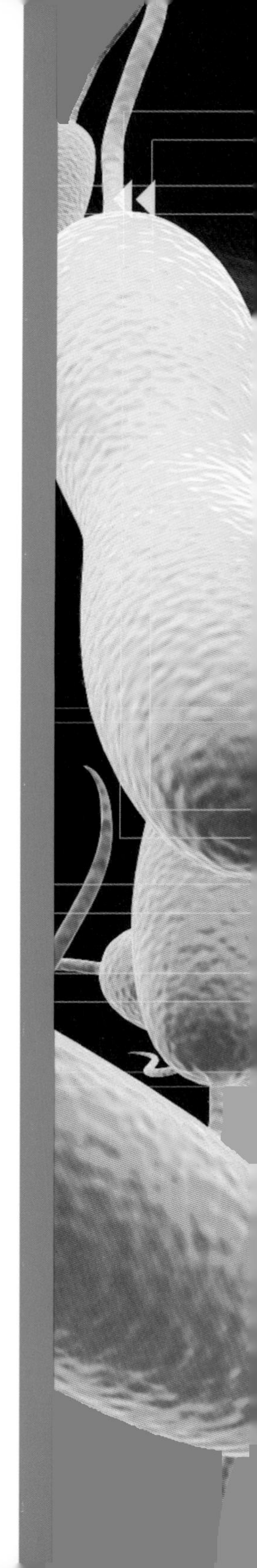

McCord Museum of Canadian History
690 Sherbrooke Street West
Montreal, QC H3A 1E9
Canada
(514) 398-7100
Web site: http://www.mccord-museum.qc.ca
The McCord Museum is devoted to preserving and studying all aspects of Canadian history. Its collections include items relating to cholera.

Public Health Agency of Canada (PHAC)
130 Colonnade Road
A.L. 6501H
Ottawa, ON K1A 0K9
Canada
Web site: http://www.phac-aspc.gc.ca
The PHAC works to improve the overall health of Canadians, as well as control diseases and respond to health emergencies.

Royal Pharmaceutical Society of Great Britain Museum
1 Lambeth High Street
London SE1 7JN
England
Phone: 020-7735-9141
Web site: http://www.rpsgb.org.uk/informationresources/museum
The museum has a collection of items relating to medicine in British history, and it provides information and a research service.

Tenement Museum
Administrative Offices
108 Orchard Street

New York, NY 10002
(212) 431-0233
Web site: http://www.tenement.org
The Tenement Museum offers tours of a tenement building, as well as information on nineteenth-century New York from an immigrant perspective.

World Health Organization (WHO)
Avenue Appia 20
1211 Geneva 27
Switzerland
Phone: 41 22 791 21 11
Web site: http://www.who.int
Operated through the United Nations, the WHO sets policies and directs research efforts on global health issues.

Web Sites

Due to the changing nature of Internet links, Rosen Publishing has developed an online list of Web sites related to the subject of this book. This site is updated regularly. Please use this link to access the list:

http://www.rosenlinks.com/epi/chol

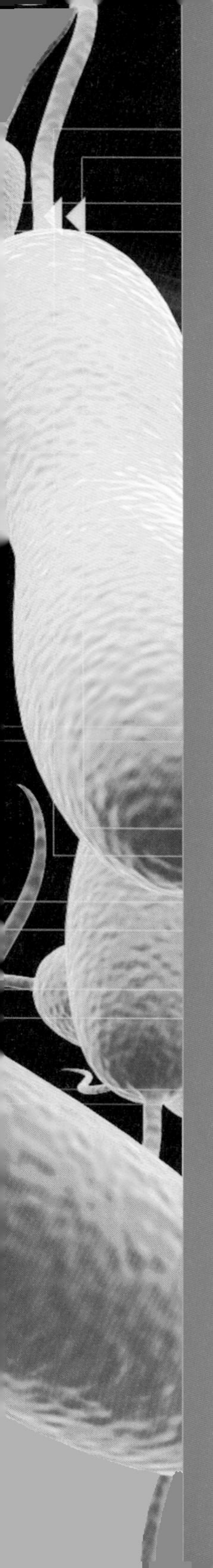

FOR FURTHER READING

Allen, Judy. *The Blue Death*. London, England: Hodder Children's Books, 2001.

Anderson, Laurie Halse. *Fever 1793*. New York, NY: Simon & Schuster Children's Publishing, 2002.

Arnold, Nick. *Deadly Diseases and Microscopic Monsters*. New York, NY: Scholastic, 2009.

Ballard, Carol. *Fighting Infectious Diseases*. Milwaukee, WI: World Almanac Library, 2007.

Barnard, Bryn. *Outbreak! Plagues That Changed History*. New York, NY: Crown Books for Young Readers, 2005.

Boring, Mel, and Leslie Dendy. *Guinea Pig Scientists*. New York, NY: Henry Holt & Co., 2005.

Coleman, William, and I. Edward Alcamo. *Cholera*. New York, NY: Facts On File, Inc., 2003.

Cooney, Caroline. *Code Orange*. New York, NY: Delacorte Books for Young Readers, 2005.

Farrell, Janette. *Invisible Enemies*. New York, NY: Farrar, Straus and Giroux, 2005.

Friedlander, Mark P., Jr. *Outbreak: Disease Detectives at Work*. Minneapolis, MN: Twenty-First Century Books, 2009.

Goldsmith, Connie. *Invisible Invaders: Dangerous Infectious Diseases*. Minneapolis, MN: Twenty-First Century Books, 2006.

Herbst, Judith. *Germ Theory*. Minneapolis, MN: Twenty-First Century Books, 2007.

Jarman, Julia. *The Sewer Sleuth*. London, England: Franklin Watts, Ltd., 2002.

Nardo, Don. *Industrial Revolution: Social and Economic Effects*. San Diego, CA: Lucent Books, 2009.

Peters, Stephanie True. *Epidemic! Cholera: Curse of the Nineteenth Century*. New York, NY: Benchmark Books, 2005.

Remington, Gwen. *Life in Victorian England*. San Diego, CA: Lucent Books, 2005.

Townsend, John. *Pox, Pus, and Plague: A History of Disease and Infection*. Chicago, IL: Raintree Publishers, 2005.

Tracy, Kathleen. *Robert Koch and the Study of Anthrax*. Hockessin, DE: Mitchell Lane Publishers, 2004.

Walker, Richard. *Epidemics and Plagues*. Boston, MA: Kingfisher Publications, 2006.

Willett, Edward. *Disease-Hunting Scientist: Careers Hunting Deadly Diseases*. Berkeley Heights, NJ: Enslow Publishers, Inc., 2009.

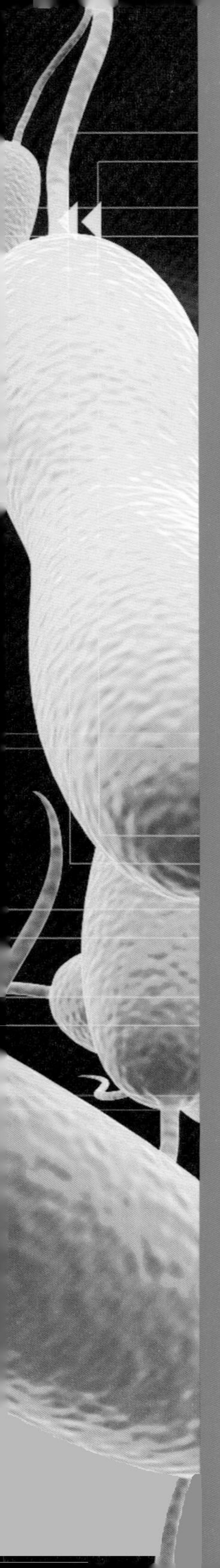

BIBLIOGRAPHY

CBC.ca. "Cholera's Seven Pandemics." December 2, 2008. Retrieved June 14, 2009. (http://www.cbc.ca/health/story/2008/05/09/f-cholera-outbreaks.html).

CUNY.edu. "Cholera in 1866." Retrieved June 13, 2009 (http://www.vny.cuny.edu/cholera/1866/cholera_1866new.html).

Delaporte, Francois. *Disease and Civilization: The Cholera in Paris, 1832*. Cambridge, MA: MIT Press, 1986.

Harvard.edu. "Cholera Epidemics in the 19th Century." Retrieved June 14, 2009 (http://ocp.hul.harvard.edu/contagion/cholera.html).

Hempel, Sandra. *The Strange Case of the Broad Street Pump.* Berkeley, CA: University of California Press, 2007.

Johnson, Steven. *The Ghost Map*. New York, NY: Riverhead Books, 2006.

Kudlick, Catherine. *Cholera in Post-Revolutionary Paris: A Cultural History*. Berkeley, CA: University of California Press, 1996.

Longmate, Norman. *King Cholera: The Biography of a Disease.* London, England: Hamish Hamilton, 1966.

Mabuse, Nkepile. "Zimbabwe Cholera Epidemic Worsening." CNN.com, February 17, 2009. Retrieved June 13, 2009 (http://www.cnn.com/2009/WORLD/africa/02/17/Zimbabwe.cholera.crisis).

McGrew, Roderick E. *Russia and the Cholera, 1823–1832.* Madison, WI: University of Wisconsin Press, 1965.

Melanson, Donald. "Dean Kamen Aims to Clean Water, Generate Electricity with Slingshot Machine." Engadget.com, April 23, 2008.

Retrieved June 22, 2009 (http://74.125.95.132/search?q=cache:TsLVsiIrnKsJ:www.engadget.com/2008/04/23/dean-kamen-aims-to-clean-water-generate-electricity-with-slings/3).

Morris, R. J. *Cholera 1832: The Social Response to an Epidemic*. New York, NY: Holmes & Meier Publishers, 1976.

Morris, Robert D. *The Blue Death*. New York, NY: HarperCollins Publishers, 2007.

Rosenberg, Charles E. *The Cholera Years: The United States in 1832, 1849, and 1866*. Chicago, IL: University of Chicago Press, 1962.

ScientificBlogging.com. "Cholera Cases in Africa Increased Due to Global Warming, Say Researchers." April 25, 2009. Retrieved June 22, 2009 (http://www.scientificblogging.com/news_articles/choera_cases_africa_increased_due_global_warming_say_researchers).

Sherman, Irwin W. *The Power of Plagues*. Washington, DC: ASM Press, 2006.

Silberner, Joanne. "Watching Peru's Oceans for Cholera Cues." NPR.org, February 25, 2008. Retrieved June 22, 2009 (http://www.npr.org/templates/story/story.php?storyId=19344123).

Snowden, Frank M. *Naples in the Time of Cholera, 1884–1911*. Cambridge, England: Cambridge University Press, 1995.

TheNakedScientists.com. "Predicting Cholera Outbreaks from Space." March 2008. Retrieved June 22, 2009 (http://www.thenakedscientists.com/HTML/content/interviews/interview/892).

Waller, John. *Einstein's Luck*. Oxford, England: Oxford University Press, 2002.

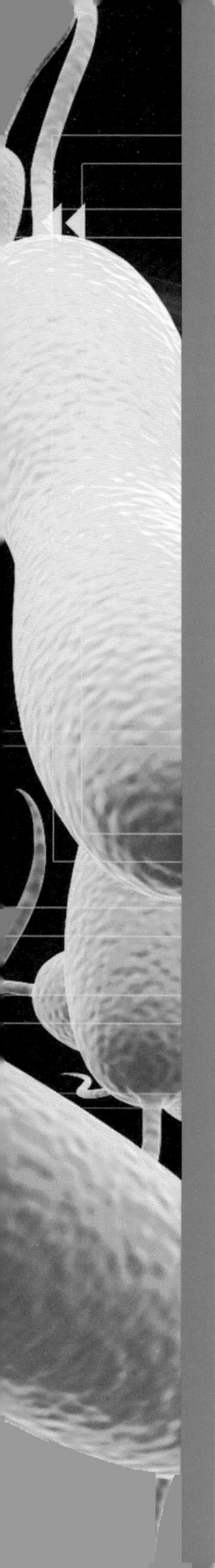

INDEX

About the Author

Diane Bailey has always been interested in gruesome diseases, with their frightening symptoms and often-fatal outcomes. While researching this book and another in the series, *The Plague*, she was fascinated to learn how diseases have changed entire societies. Bailey lives in Kansas and writes on a variety of nonfiction topics.

Photo Credits

Cover, pp. 7, 15, 24, 34, 42, 52, 60, 69, 71, 74, 76, 78 Shutterstock.com; pp. 4–5, 36–37 Mansell/Time & Life Pictures/Getty Images; p. 9 HIP/Art Resource, NY; pp. 10–11 Pedro Ugarte/AFP/Getty Images; p.13 General Photographic Agency/Getty Images; p. 16 Private Collection/Giraudon/ The Bridgeman Art Library; pp. 18–19 MPI/Getty Images; pp. 22–23 © Trustees of the Watts Gallery, Compton, Surrey,UK/The Bridgeman Art Library; p. 25 © Courtesy of the Warden and Scholars of New College, Oxford/The Bridgeman Art Library; pp. 28–29, 57 Hulton Archive/Getty Images; pp. 30–31 Josef Mensing Gallery, Hamm-Rhynern, Germany/ The Bridgeman Art Library; p. 35 Museé de la Ville de Paris, Museé Carnavalet, Paris, France/Giraudon/The Bridgeman Art library; p. 40 Bildarchiv Preussischer Kulturbesitz/Art Resource, NY; pp. 43, 44–45, 47, 49 History of Medicine/NLM; p. 53 Hans Gelderblom/Stone/Getty Images; pp. 54–55 CDC; p. 58 © World History/Topham/The Image Works; p. 61 Jaime Razuri/AFP/Getty Images; pp. 62–63 Malcolm Linton/Liaison/Getty Images; pp. 66–67 Desmond Kwande/AFP/Getty Images.

Designer: Sam Zavieh; Editor: Bethany Bryan;
Photo Researcher: Amy Feinberg